Fast Facts for Healthcare
Professionals

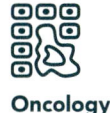

Oncology

Neuroblastoma

Jennifer Foster MD, MPH
Cancer and Hematology Center
Texas Children's Hospital
Department of Pediatrics
Section of Hematology and Oncology
Baylor College of Medicine
Houston, Texas, USA

Michelle Choe MD
Assistant Professor
Clinical Research Division
Fred Hutchinson Cancer Center
Department of Pediatrics
University of Washington
Hematology/Oncology/Bone marrow transplantation
Seattle Children's Hospital
Seattle, Washington, USA

Erika A Newman MD
Michael W Mulholland Professor of Surgery
Chief, Section of Pediatric Surgery
Department of Surgery
C. S. Mott Children's Hospital
University of Michigan
Ann Arbor, Michigan, USA

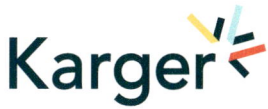

HEALTHCARE

Fast Facts: Neuroblastoma
First published 2025

Text © 2025 Jennifer Foster, Michelle Choe, Erika A Newman
© 2025 in this edition S. Karger Publishers Ltd

S. Karger Publishers Ltd, Merchant House, 5 East St. Helen Street, Abingdon, Oxford OX14 5EG, UK

Book orders can be placed by telephone or email, or via the website.
Please telephone +41 61 306 1440 or email orders@karger.com
To order via the website, please go to karger.com

Fast Facts is a trademark of S. Karger Publishers Ltd.

All rights reserved. No part of this publication may be reproduced, stored in a retrieval system, or transmitted in any form or by any means, electronic, mechanical, photocopying, recording or otherwise, without the express permission of the publisher.

The rights of Jennifer Foster, Michelle Choe and Erika A Newman to be identified as the authors of this work have been asserted in accordance with the Copyright, Designs & Patents Act 1988 Sections 77 and 78.

The publisher and the authors have made every effort to ensure the accuracy of this book, but cannot accept responsibility for any errors or omissions.

For all drugs, please consult the product labeling approved in your country for prescribing information.

Registered names, trademarks, etc. used in this book, even when not marked as such, are not to be considered unprotected by law.

A CIP record for this title is available from the British Library.

ISBN 978-3-318-06512-1

Foster J (Jennifer)
Fast Facts: Neuroblastoma/
Jennifer Foster, Michelle Choe, Erika A Newman

Medical illustrations by Graeme Chambers, Belfast, UK.
Typesetting by Amnet, Chennai, India.
Printed in the UK with XPedient.

An independent publication developed by S. Karger Publishers Ltd and provided as a service to medicine. Supported by an educational grant from Y-mAbs Therapeutics.

List of abbreviations	5
Introduction	7
Epidemiology and etiology	9
Pathogenesis	17
Diagnosis	27
Staging and risk stratification	41
Management	51
Health disparities	75
Future directions and unmet needs	81
Survivorship	95
Useful resources	105
Index	107

List of abbreviations

ADP: adenosine diphosphate

ALK: anaplastic lymphoma kinase

ALT: alternative lengthening of telomeres

ASCT: autologous stem cell transplant

ATP: adenosine triphosphate

CAR T cell: chimeric antigen receptor T cell

CBC: complete blood count

CCG: Children's Cancer Group

CCSS: Childhood Cancer Survivor Study

CEM: carboplatin, etoposide and melphalan

CI: confidence interval

CILP: cumulative incidence of local progression

CNS: central nervous system

CNV: copy number variation

COG: Children's Oncology Group

CT: computed tomography

ctDNA: circulating tumor DNA

ddPCR: digital droplet polymerase chain reaction

DNA: deoxyribonucleic acid

EFS: event-free survival

FDA: Food and Drug Administration

FISH: fluorescence in-situ hybridization

GM-CSF: granulocyte-macrophage colony-stimulating factor

GTR: gross total resection

HDAC: histone deacetylase

HDI: human development index

HR: hazard ratio

IDRF: image-defined risk factor

IL-2: interleukin-2

INRG: International Neuroblastoma Risk Group

INRGSS: International Neuroblastoma Risk Group Staging System

INSS: International Neuroblastoma Staging System

L1CAM: L1 cell adhesion molecule

lncRNA: long non-coding RNA

LOH: loss-of-heterozygosity

mAb: monoclonal antibody

MAPK: mitogen-activated protein kinase

MIBG: meta-iodobenzylguanidine (imaging)

miR: microRNA

MRI: magnetic resonance imaging

MYC-N: myelocytomatosis viral-related oncogene, neuroblastoma (encoded by *MYCN*)

NANT: New Approaches to Neuroblastoma Therapy (consortium)

NGF: nerve growth factor

NK: natural killer (T cells)

NTRK: neurotrophic receptor tyrosine kinase

OMAS: opsoclonus-myoclonus-ataxia syndrome

ORR: overall response rate

OS: overall survival

PEP-CTN: The Pediatric Early Phase Clinical Trials Network

PHOX2A/B: paired-like homeobox 2 A/B

PI3K: phosphoinositide 3-kinase

RNA: ribonucleic acid

ROS1: c-ros oncogene 1

SCA: segmental chromosome aberration

SEER: Surveillance, Epidemiology, and End Results

SES: socioeconomic status

SIOP: International Society of Paediatric Oncology

SIOPEN: International Society of Paediatric Oncology European Neuroblastoma Group

SNP: single-nucleotide polymorphism

TBI: total body irradiation

VEGF: vascular endothelial growth factor

VIP: vasoactive intestinal peptide

Introduction

Neuroblastoma is the most common extracranial solid tumor in children, with the highest incidence in children aged under 5 years. It is a fascinating disease that manifests in heterogeneous ways. It is a challenging disease to treat, and advances in therapy have led to improvements in survival rates.

Low- and intermediate-risk tumors carry a 5-year survival rate of over 90%, while the 5-year survival rate for high-risk disease is only around 50%. As our understanding of this disease deepens, therapy for aggressive disease will continue to advance, resulting in improved survival possibilities.

In *Fast Facts: Neuroblastoma*, we review the epidemiology and what is understood thus far about the pathogenesis of neuroblastoma. We then dive into the various ways in which neuroblastoma may present and outline the diagnostic studies needed to complete workup. We review prognostic factors and disease risk stratification, followed by a comprehensive overview of treatment regimens for low-, intermediate- and high-risk disease. Later chapters discuss health disparities, new treatment modalities under study, late effects of treatment and survivorship. This concise, yet comprehensive, overview of neuroblastoma is designed for medical students, primary care providers, hematology, oncology and surgical trainees, and nurses. We hope that this book will serve as a valuable resource and guide.

1 Epidemiology and etiology

Oncology

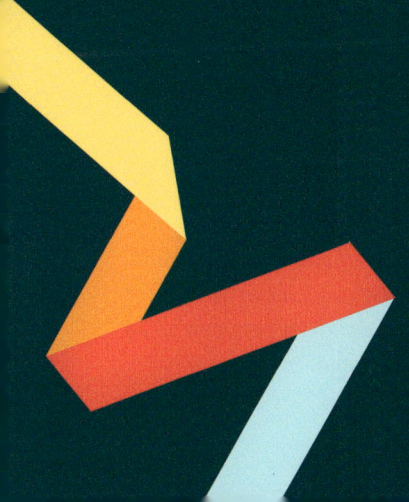

HEALTHCARE

Epidemiology

Prevalence. Neuroblastoma is the third most common childhood cancer worldwide, accounting for approximately 10% of all pediatric cancers and up to 15% of all cancer deaths in children.[1] It is also the most common extracranial solid tumor in children, and is by far the most common cancer in children aged under 1 year.[2,3] In the USA, neuroblastoma accounts for around 6% of cancers in patients aged up to and including 14 years, and less than 1% in those aged between 15 and 19 years.[4] It represents approximately 97% of all neuroblastic tumors.[5]

Approximately 700–800 new cases of neuroblastoma are diagnosed each year in the USA, a number that has been fairly stable over the last few decades.[2] Although neuroblastoma is occasionally detected by ultrasound before birth, the mean age of children at the time of diagnosis is 1–2 years (median 19 months). Around 40% of diagnoses occur before 3 months of age and around 90% by 5 years.[3] It is rare in individuals aged 10 years and older.[2] An analysis of the US-based Surveillance, Epidemiology, and End Results (SEER) database (from 1973 to 2007) found that around 6% of all patients with neuroblastoma were aged 20 years and older at diagnosis, and that only 1% were aged 60 years or older.[6]

Incidence of neuroblastoma in the USA is 4.9 cases per million individuals overall and 11–13 cases per million children aged under 15 years.[3] Incidence decreases with each consecutive year up to age 10 years. The most recent SEER data for incidence rates of neuroblastoma and ganglioneuroblastoma, age-adjusted to the 2000 US standard population, are shown in Figure 1.1. The data shown correspond to broader age groups (10.5 and 8.1 cases per million individuals per year for ages 0–14 and 0–19 years, respectively).[7] Recent analysis of the SEER program database found that, between 1975 and 2013, incidence of neuroblastoma in children aged 14 years or younger had increased.[3]

In Europe, the age-adjusted incidence rates of neuroblastoma between 1988 and 1997 were estimated to be 10.9 cases per million children and 52.6 cases per million infants aged 0–12 months. Incidence increased from 8.4 cases per million children between 1978 and 1982 to 11.6 cases per million children between 1993 and 1997,

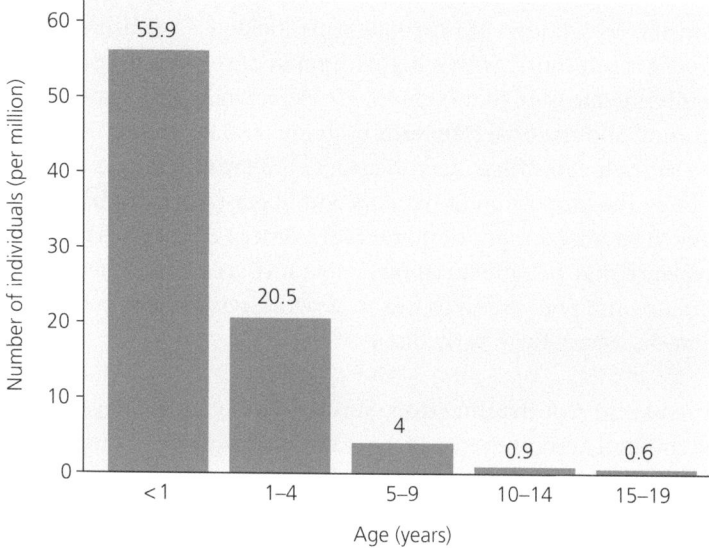

Figure 1.1 The most recent SEER data for incidence rates of neuroblastoma and ganglioneuroblastoma per million individuals per year, age-adjusted to the 2000 US standard population.[7]

believed to be partly due to a degree of overdiagnosis in children aged under 2 years.[8]

Sex and ethnicity. Incidence of neuroblastoma is lower in Black children than White children and other ethnic groups. It is slightly higher in boys, with a male-to-female ratio of 1.2:1.[9]

Overdiagnosis effects have been found to result from screening programs for neuroblastoma. When a national screening program was stopped in Japan in 2003, a marked decrease in incidence was observed that brought it in line with incidence reported in the USA.[10] The program was judged to have resulted in overdiagnosis because mortality did not change.[11] Similar overdiagnosis effects have been reported by studies of screening programs for neuroblastoma conducted in parts of Canada and Germany.[12,13]

Geographic differences in neuroblastoma incidence are often regarded to be negligible.[1] However, some variations exist and a link with the level of socioeconomic development has been noted. Neuroblastoma is relatively rare in many low- and middle-income countries. A high level of neuroblastoma incidence has been shown to correlate significantly with a higher human development index (HDI), a composite measure that includes life expectancy, anticipated education and national standards of living ($r=0.81$; $p<0.001$).[14]

In sub-Saharan Africa, neuroblastoma is relatively uncommon, although the proportion of patients with metastatic neuroblastoma seems to be higher than is reported for Western countries. Here, prevalence may be influenced by factors such as a lack of health insurance and poor access to health services, resulting in low rates of diagnosis, especially in early disease.[15]

Survival and risk stratification. Survival rates vary with age, such that children aged under 1 year at diagnosis have significantly greater 5-year survival than those diagnosed when older.[5] Risk stratification has uncovered widely divergent outcomes, ranging from cure in more than 90% of patients with low- and intermediate-risk disease to less than 50% for those with high-risk disease (see Chapter 4).

In recent decades, survival rates have improved with the development of effective therapies and treatment regimens based on risk stratification, which utilize combinations of prognostic clinical and biological markers. Between 1975 and 2013, there was a trend for improved overall survival (OS) in all age groups in the USA, despite an increase in children presenting at later stages of disease.[3]

In a Europe-wide study covering the years 1978–1997, 5-year survival was 59% overall, ranging from 47% in Eastern Europe to 67% in Western Europe. Overall, 5-year survival improved from 37% in 1978–1982 to 66% in 1993–1997.[8] A degree of overdiagnosis in children aged under 2 years was judged, in part, to explain the increase in survival. However, improved survival of older children (aged 2–14 years), from 21% to 45%, was deemed to be largely due to improved therapy.[8]

In a population-based study in the USA, it was found that most patients with newly diagnosed, histologically confirmed neuroblastoma in 2010 and 2011 were enrolled in clinical trials.[16] Using the Children's Oncology Group (COG) system of three-level (low, intermediate and high) neuroblastoma risk classification (see Chapter 4), all low-risk patients received surgery or observation, most intermediate-risk patients (81%) received a chemotherapy regimen and high-risk patients received extensive, multimodal treatment. Low- and intermediate-risk patients were found to have excellent survival rates, while the estimated 5-year survival rate for high-risk patients was 45%. This was a substantial improvement on the 29% reported for those diagnosed between 1990 and 1994, but comparable to the 5-year survival rate of 50% reported for patients diagnosed between 2005 and 2010.[16] Studies in Spain and Italy have also found that survival rates are better within the strict framework of clinical trials, and that prompt identification and risk stratification of *MYCN* (encodes MYC-N [myelocytomatosis viral-related oncogene, neuroblastoma]) amplification status improves survival.[17]

Racial and ethnic disparities in risk and survival were demonstrated among over 3500 patients enrolled in the COG neuroblastoma biology study in the USA, with Black and Native American children having greater prevalence of high-risk disease than White children ($p<0.001$ and $p=0.04$, respectively) and significantly lower event-free survival (EFS) ($p=0.01$ and $p=0.002$, respectively). Examination of EFS among high-risk patients who remained event free for at least 2 years showed increased prevalence of late-occurring events among Black children compared with White children (see Chapter 6 for more on outcome disparities).[18]

Etiology

The underlying etiology of most neuroblastoma tumors remains unknown. The majority occur in isolation, suggesting that rates of oncogenic germline mutations are low in patients with neuroblastoma.

Environmental factors such as maternal medication use, childhood infections, and exposure to metals such as chromium and nickel have been suggested to be possible causes, but no direct links have been established.[1] As noted earlier in this chapter, increasing incidence of neuroblastoma has been shown to correlate significantly with increasing HDI. It is thought that the effects of perinatal and early life environmental exposures, combined with those of germline predisposition, may be responsible.[14]

Genetic predisposition occurs in approximately 1–2% of neuroblastoma cases, with autosomal dominance with incomplete penetrance (~65%) being the mode of inheritance.

Germline mutations in the *ALK* gene account for most familial cases of neuroblastoma,[19] but mutations in *PHOX2B* (associated with Hirschsprung disease and central hypoventilation syndrome) and *KIF1B* have also been identified in patients with genetically inherited neuroblastoma.[1,5] Familial neuroblastoma cases typically present with multifocal or bilateral adrenal primary tumors and are diagnosed at a median age of 9 months.[1]

Cancer predisposition syndromes, such as Li-Fraumeni syndrome, RASopathies and mutations in *SDHB* may also cause a slight increase in the risk of neuroblastoma.[10]

Karyotypic abnormalities associated with congenital neuroblastoma have been reported, including partial trisomy of 2p, which leads to triplication of the *MYCN* region of 2p24.3 in germline cells,[20] and de novo 14q23.1–q23.3 microdeletion.[21]

Associations with other diseases have been identified. Neurocristopathies such as Hirschsprung disease and central hypoventilation syndrome are known to be associated with neuroblastoma, although the underlying etiologies of these associations are not understood. There have also been reports of neuroblastoma in patients with neurofibromatosis, although whether germline *NF1* mutations play a role in the etiology of neuroblastoma is unknown.[1]

Key points – epidemiology and etiology

- Neuroblastoma is the most common extracranial solid tumor in children worldwide, and by far the most common cancer in those aged 1 year and under.
- The incidence of neuroblastoma is 11–13 cases per million children aged under 15 years.
- Incidence is slightly higher in males than females, and the prevalence of high-risk disease is greater in Black and Native American children than in White children.
- The etiology of most neuroblastoma tumors remains unknown, although an underlying familial genetic predisposition occurs in 1–2% of neuroblastoma cases.

References

1. Whittle SB, Smith V, Doherty E et al. Overview and recent advances in the treatment of neuroblastoma. *Expert Rev Anticancer Ther* 2017;17:369–86.
2. American Cancer Society. *Key Statistics About Neuroblastoma.* American Cancer Society, 2021. cancer.org/cancer/neuroblastoma/about/key-statistics.html, last accessed 10 May 2022.
3. Yan P, Qi F, Bian L et al. Comparison of incidence and outcomes of neuroblastoma in children, adolescents, and adults in the United States: a Surveillance, Epidemiology, and End Results (SEER) program population study. *Med Sci Monit* 2020;26:e927218.
4. Siegel RL, Miller KD, Fuchs HE, Jemal A. Cancer statistics, 2021. *CA Cancer J Clin* 2021;71:7–33.
5. Swift CC, Eklund MJ, Kraveka JM, Alazraki AL. Updates in diagnosis, management, and treatment of neuroblastoma. *Radiographics* 2018;38:566–80.
6. Rogowitz E, Babiker HM, Kanaan M et al. Neuroblastoma of the elderly, an oncologist's nightmare: case presentation, literature review and SEER database analysis. *Exp Hematol Oncol* 2014;30:20.
7. Howlader N, Noone AM, Krapcho M et al. *SEER Cancer Statistics Review, 1975–2018.* National Cancer Institute, 2021. seer.cancer.gov/csr/1975_2018/, last accessed 10 May 2022.
8. Spix C, Pastore G, Sankila R et al. Neuroblastoma incidence and survival in European children (1978–1997): report from the Automated Childhood Cancer Information System project. *Eur J Cancer* 2006;42:2081–91.
9. Lacayo NJ. *Pediatric Neuroblastoma.* Medscape, 2021. emedicine.medscape.com/article/988284-overview#a6, last accessed 10 May 2022.
10. Nakagawara A, Li Y, Izumi H et al. Neuroblastoma. *Jpn J Clin Oncol* 2018;48:214–41.
11. Shinagawa T, Kitamura T, Katanoda K et al. The incidence and mortality rates of neuroblastoma cases before and after the cessation of the mass screening program in Japan: a descriptive study. *Int J Cancer* 2017;140:618–25.
12. Schilling FH, Spix C, Berthold F et al. Neuroblastoma screening at one year of age. *N Engl J Med* 2002;346:1047–53.
13. Woods WG, Gao RN, Shuster JJ et al. Screening of infants and mortality due to neuroblastoma. *N Engl J Med* 2002;346:1041–6.
14. Kamihara J, Ma C, Fuentes Alabi SL et al. Socioeconomic status and global variations in the incidence of neuroblastoma: call for support of population-based cancer registries in low-middle-income countries. *Pediatr Blood Cancer* 2017;64:321–3.

15. Traoré F, Eshun F, Togo B et al. Neuroblastoma in Africa: a survey by the Franco-African Pediatric Oncology Group. *J Glob Oncol* 2016;2:169–73.
16. Coughlan D, Gianferante M, Lynch CF et al. Treatment and survival of childhood neuroblastoma: evidence from a population-based study in the United States. *Pediatr Hematol Oncol* 2017;34:320–30.
17. Di Cataldo A, Agodi A, Balaguer J et al. Metastatic neuroblastoma in infants: are survival rates excellent only within the stringent framework of clinical trials? *Clin Transl Oncol* 2017;19:76–83.
18. Henderson TO, Bhatia S, Pinto N et al. Racial and ethnic disparities in risk and survival in children with neuroblastoma: a Children's Oncology Group study. *J Clin Oncol* 2011;29:76–82.
19. Matthay KK, Maris JM, Schleiermacher G et al. Neuroblastoma. *Nat Rev Dis Primers* 2016;2:16078.
20. Van Mater D, Knelson EH, Kaiser-Rogers KA, Armstrong MB. Neuroblastoma in a pediatric patient with a microduplication of 2p involving the MYCN locus. *Am J Med Genet A* 2013; 161A:605–10.
21. Lehalle D, Sanlaville D, Guimier A et al. Multiple congenital anomalies-intellectual disability (MCA-ID) and neuroblastoma in a patient harboring a de novo 14q23.1q23.3 deletion. *Am J Med Genet A* 2014;164A:1310–7.

2 Pathogenesis

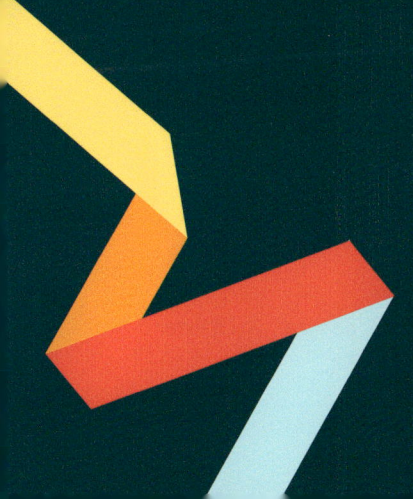

Neuroblastomas can arise at any location in the sympathetic nervous system. Most tumors occur in the abdomen, with the majority arising in the adrenal medulla (Figure 2.1).[1,2] Among patients with neuroblastoma, the most common primary tumor sites are adrenal (47%), abdominal/retroperitoneal (24%), thoracic (15%), pelvic (3%) and neck (3%),[3] while primary CNS neuroblastoma has been reported in a small number of case studies.[4] Common sites of metastasis include distant lymph nodes, bone, bone marrow and liver.[1,2]

Tumor biology

Neuroblastoma arises from cells that normally form the embryonic structure known as the neural crest. Normal development of the neural crest depends on multipotent and migratory cell populations that are capable of differentiating into diverse cell lineages, including mature peripheral neural tissues. During this process, many embryonic neurons are thought to undergo apoptosis when nerve

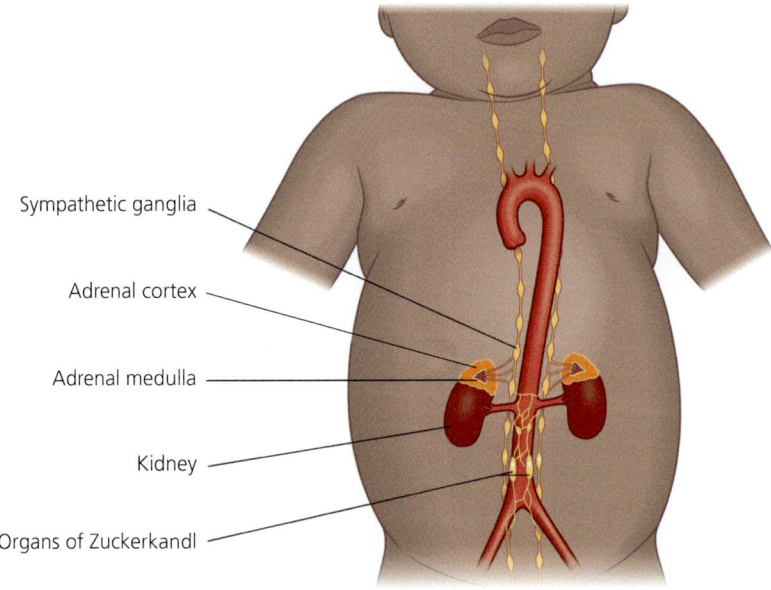

Figure 2.1 Anatomic distribution of the sympathetic ganglia, which extend from the neck to the pelvic region, and adrenal medulla.

growth factor (NGF; also known as neural growth factor) becomes limiting for their survival during development.[5] Neuroblastoma is thought to arise only from the precursor cells of the sympathoadrenal lineage, and it is assumed that the multipotent neural crest cells accumulate mutations and epigenetic changes that contribute to tumorigenesis via the failure of ligand–receptor signaling mechanisms that direct transcription factors involved in normal morphological differentiation (Table 2.1).[6,7] Although the details of this process are poorly understood, NGF (one of four neurotrophins in humans)

TABLE 2.1

Involvement of signaling pathways in neural crest cell development and the formation of tumor-initiating neuroblastoma cancer stem cells

Stage of differentiation	Neural crest development	Pathogenesis of neuroblastoma
Neural tube → neural plate border	Neural crest induction: BMP, Wnt/Fzd, fibroblast growth factor/STAT3, notch/delta	BMP, Wnt
Neural plate border → premigratory neural crest	Neural crest speciation: c-Myc, Id3 (early onset), SOX9/10, FOXD3, SNAIL2, Twist1	c-Myc, MYC-N, FOXD3, Twist1 (direct target of MYC-N)
Premigratory → postmigratory neural crest	Delamination/EMT: type II cadherins, MMPs, ADAM1, β1 integrin	EMT pathway genes
Postmigratory neural crest → sympathoadrenal progenitors	Sympathoadrenal speciation: PHOX2A/B, ASCL1, HAND2, GATA2/3	PHOX2B

ADAM1, disintegrin and metalloproteinase domain-containing protein 1; ASCL1, Achaete-Scute family BHLH transcription factor 1; BMP, bone morphogenetic protein; EMT, epithelial–mesenchymal transition; FOXD3, forkhead box D3; Fzd, Frizzled; GATA2/3, GATA-binding protein 2/3; HAND2, heart and neural crest derivatives expressed 2; Id3, inhibitor of DNA binding 3; MMP, matrix metalloproteinase; PHOX2A/B, paired-like homeobox 2 A/B; SNAIL2, snail family transcriptional repressor 2; SOX9/10, SRY-box transcription factor 9/10; STAT3, signal transducer and activator of transcription 3; Twist1, twist family BHLH transcription factor 1. Adapted from Tomolonis et al. 2018.[7]

and its receptor, neurotrophic receptor tyrosine kinase (NTRK) 1, are known to play a key role in normal development and can become dysregulated.[8]

Spontaneous regression is a feature of many neuroblastomas, to an almost unique extent among human cancers, and can occur without therapy at primary or metastatic tumor sites. It is most apparent in infants with stage MS disease (age ≤ 18 months and usually with small abdominal primary tumors, but also with metastases to the liver, skin and bone marrow; see Chapter 4). The underlying mechanisms of spontaneous regression are not well characterized but are thought to involve apoptosis that may result from tumor cells being deprived of NGF.[8] Involvement of loss of telomerase activity, epigenetic regulation and immune responses has also been proposed.[9]

To date, no single biological or genetic marker has been proved to be useful for accurate diagnosis of this complex disease, although several oncogenic drivers of malignancy are known. Neuroblastic tumors are variable in their behavior, have different possible clinical courses (from metastatic spread to spontaneous regression) and their genetic makeup is similarly diverse.[1]

Amplification of MYC-N, a transcription factor that activates or represses gene transcription through direct DNA binding as well as indirect protein–protein interaction mechanisms, is involved in controlling multiple essential cellular processes, including the cell cycle, apoptosis and differentiation.[6] It is essential in normal brain development and is expressed in nervous system and mesenchymal tissues during stages of embryogenesis. MYC-N plays a key role in neuroblastoma pathogenesis and in other aggressive tumors, and its expression is normally very low in non-cancerous adult tissues.[6] MYC-N expression levels are high in a subset of poorly differentiated aggressive neuroblastomas but lower in others, suggesting that MYC-N activation is not the only mechanism that initiates tumorigenesis.[10]

Anaplastic lymphoma kinase (ALK) and paired-like homeobox 2B (PHOX2B) are also thought to play key roles in pathogenesis. They are upregulated in some neuroblastomas and their genes can be mutated in familial neuroblastoma (see page 23).

Anaplastic lymphoma kinase, an orphan receptor tyrosine kinase normally expressed only in the developing embryonic and neonatal brain, plays a role by upregulating oncogenic downstream signaling pathways including the phosphoinositide 3-kinase (PI3K) pathway, the RAS/MAPK (mitogen-activated protein kinase) pathway and the RET pathway. About one-half of all neuroblastoma samples show ALK positivity in most (>50%) tumor cells, and ALK positivity demonstrated by immunohistochemistry is an independent indicator of poor prognosis.[11]

Paired-like homeobox 2B functions as a transcription factor and is normally involved in the regulation of the differentiation program of the sympathetic nervous system.[6] PHOX2B positivity, defined as the presence of nuclear immunoreactivity in at least 5% of cells, has been shown to be present in 94% of peripheral neuroblastic tumors in children but consistently absent in non-peripheral ones. It can distinguish neuroblastoma from 'histological mimics' such as Wilms tumor, Ewing sarcoma and capicua transcriptional repressor (CIC)-rearranged round cell sarcoma.[12]

Genetics

Several karyotypic and genetic types contribute to pathogenesis (as well as risk classification in the clinic, where molecular typing is now routine). Karyotype abnormalities and *MYCN* gene amplification have been associated with neuroblastoma prognosis for over 20 years.

Karyotype and chromosome abnormalities

Aneuploidy (the presence of ≥1 extra chromosome or the absence of ≥1 chromosome) is common in neuroblastoma. In patients aged 1 year or younger with localized disease, a hyperdiploid or near-triploid karyotype (caused by mitotic dysfunction where whole chromosomes are gained) is associated with very good prognosis. However, a near-diploid or near-tetraploid karyotype in patients aged 1 year or older is associated with advanced stage and rapidly progressive disease.

Polyploidy can be assessed (although crudely) by tumor cell DNA content and indexed to normal cells (normal content=1), such that neuroblastomas with higher levels of DNA content (>1 or hyperdiploid) are associated with lower tumor stage and improved outcomes in children aged under 18 months.[2] Tumor cell ploidy is less useful as a prognostic indicator in older children compared with younger children.

Copy number variations and segmental chromosome aberrations are also a feature of advanced stage and rapidly progressive disease in patients aged 1 year or older. Common copy number variations (CNVs) include deletions (also known as allelic losses or loss-of-heterozygosity [LOH]) of 1p, 3p, 4p, 6q, 11q and 14q, and gains of 1q, 2p and 17q.[2,6] Early research showed that some deletions (such as 11q) showed a correlation with regional and metastatic disease, while others (such as 14q) were less informative.[13] Research is under way to identify specific genes of importance in deleted regions.

Overall genomic karyotyping, tested using array-based comparative genomic hybridization, has provided further insights into the roles of CNVs in neuroblastoma.[14] Our understanding of the relationship of CNVs with outcome can be summarized as:
- tumors with only whole-chromosome CNVs are associated with excellent survival[14]
- segmental chromosome aberrations (SCAs) may be associated with response,[15] risk of relapse and survival, and aid in risk stratification.[14,16]

Other genetic drivers of neuroblastoma

MYCN amplification. Approximately 20% of patients with neuroblastoma show amplification of the *MYCN* locus, which is located on chromosome 2 and can be detected by fluorescence in-situ hybridization (FISH) analysis of tumor tissue.[6] Most groups define 'amplification' as greater than four times the number of *MYCN* copy genes when compared with a control 2p probe. Most tumors with *MYCN* amplification have 50–400 copies per cell, and the degree of amplification correlates strongly with advanced disease stage, rapid tumor progression and a poorer prognosis, with significantly worse EFS and OS rates.[2,17]

TERT rearrangements, affecting telomerase activation and telomere length (a useful marker of prognosis of various cancers), are seen in ~30% of high-risk neuroblastomas and are associated with poor prognosis. They seem to be mutually exclusive with *MYCN* amplification or *ATRX* mutation.[18]

Somatic point mutations are not as common in neuroblastoma as other tumors, and point mutations or deletions have been characterized in a few important genes. Some of these have high rates of detection after relapse.

ALK germline mutations have been implicated as a prominent cause of most cases of familial neuroblastoma. Similar mutations in *ALK* are somatically acquired in 7–12% of non-familial cases of neuroblastoma.[6,19] Over 35 different mutations in *ALK* have been reported, most being point mutations in one of three residues in the tyrosine-kinase domain (F1174, F1245 or R1275) that result in constitutive ALK activation.[9] The *ALK* gene is amplified in 2–3% of non-familial neuroblastoma tumors and, because its chromosomal location (2p23) is close to that of *MYCN*, *ALK* can sometimes be coamplified with *MYCN*.[6]

In a large study of 240 patients with neuroblastoma aged older than 18 months at diagnosis with metastatic (stage M; see Chapter 4) disease, of several genes found to be mutated, *ALK* was the only one that was associated with clinical outcome, with patients with *ALK* mutation having decreased OS probability ($p<0.05$). Interestingly, activating *ALK* variants were not found to be associated with *MYCN* amplification in this study.[19]

ATRX loss-of-function mutations (mostly multiexon deletions) were found in 9.6% of patients with neuroblastoma aged older than 18 months at diagnosis with metastatic (stage M; see Chapter 4) disease. Mutations in *ATRX* and *MYCN* (including amplification) are not seen together and seem to be mutually exclusive; however, *ATRX* mutations and deletions have been shown to be associated with alternative lengthening of telomeres (ALT).[18] *ATRX* mutations are more common in older than younger children.[19]

MYCN point mutations have been found in 1.7% of patients with neuroblastoma aged older than 18 months at diagnosis with metastatic (stage 4; see Chapter 4) disease.[19]

PTNP11 (also known as *Shp-2*, *Syp*, *PTP2C* or *593aa*) functions downstream of several growth factor receptors and plays a role in cell spreading and migration. It is mutated in 2.9% of cases of neuroblastoma in patients aged older than 18 months at diagnosis with metastatic (stage 4; see Chapter 4) disease.[19] Mutations in *PTPN11*, reported in some hematologic malignancies but otherwise rare in other cancers, are also seen in Noonan syndrome, which is characterized by multiple congenital anomalies.[20]

NRAS-activating mutations and activating mutations in other components of the MAPK pathway were recently described as being present at low levels (3%) at diagnosis but in a high proportion (around 78%) of neuroblastoma tumors at relapse; some of the mutations were novel while others were clonally enriched at relapse.[18] *NRAS* mutations are seen at low rates (0.83%) in older children (age >18 months) at diagnosis.[19]

TP53 is mutated in around 2% of neuroblastomas at presentation. Mutations can be acquired during treatment and *TP53* mutations are detected in 15% of neuroblastomas at relapse.[18]

Other genes found to be mutated at low frequencies in older children (age >18 months) at diagnosis are *OR5T1* and *PDE6G*, found in 1.25% and 0.83% of neuroblastomas, respectively.[19]

Key points – pathogenesis

- Neuroblastoma can arise at any location in the sympathetic nervous system, but the most common primary tumor site is the adrenal medulla. Common sites of metastasis include the distant lymph nodes, bone, bone marrow and liver.
- Spontaneous regression can occur without therapy in primary or metastatic tumor sites, and is most apparent in infants with stage MS disease (see Chapter 4).
- ALK and PHOX2B are often overexpressed in neuroblastomas and can be used as histological markers to detect neuroblastoma cells in biopsies. Mutations in *ALK* are associated with decreased OS.
- Chromosome CNV provides valuable prognostic information, such that tumors with only whole-chromosome CNVs are associated with excellent survival, while certain SCAs can be associated with higher-risk disease.
- The degree of *MYCN* amplification strongly correlates with advanced disease stage, poor prognosis and reduced OS.
- Somatic point mutations are not as common in neuroblastoma as in other tumors, but point mutations or deletions have been characterized in a few important genes.

References

1. Lonergan GJ, Schwab CM, Suarez ES, Carlson CL. Neuroblastoma, ganglioneuroblastoma, and ganglioneuroma: radiologic-pathologic correlation. *Radiographics* 2002;22:911–34.
2. Swift CC, Eklund MJ, Kraveka JM et al. Updates in diagnosis, management, and treatment of neuroblastoma. *Radiographics* 2018;38:566–80.
3. Vo KT, Matthay KK, Neuhaus J et al. Clinical, biologic, and prognostic differences on the basis of primary tumor site in neuroblastoma: a report from the international neuroblastoma risk group project. *J Clin Oncol* 2014; 32:3169–76.
4. Mishra A, Beniwal M, Nandeesh BN et al. Primary pediatric intracranial neuroblastoma: a report of two cases. *J Pediatr Neurosci* 2018;13:366–70.
5. Bernards R. Unlikely suspects identified in neuroblastoma conspiracy. *Cancer Discov* 2014;4:392–3.
6. Nakagawara A, Li Y, Izumi H et al. Neuroblastoma. *Jpn J Clin Oncol* 2018;48:214–41.
7. Tomolonis JA, Agarwal S, Shohet JM. Neuroblastoma pathogenesis: deregulation of embryonic neural crest development. *Cell Tissue Res* 2018;372:245–62.
8. Aygun N. Biological and genetic features of neuroblastoma and their clinical importance. *Curr Pediatr Rev* 2018;14:73–90.
9. Johnsen JI, Dyberg C, Wickström M. Neuroblastoma—a neural crest derived embryonal malignancy. *Front Mol Neurosci* 2019;12:9.
10. Louis CU, Shohet JM. Neuroblastoma: molecular pathogenesis and therapy. *Annu Rev Med* 2015;66:49–63.
11. Duijkers FAM, Gaal J, Meijerink JPP et al. High anaplastic lymphoma kinase immunohistochemical staining in neuroblastoma and ganglioneuroblastoma is an independent predictor of poor outcome. *Am J Pathol* 2012;180:1223–31.
12. Hung YP, Lee JP, Bellizzi AM, Hornick JL. PHOX2B reliably distinguishes neuroblastoma among small round blue cell tumours. *Histopathology* 2017;71:786–94.
13. Srivatsan ES, Ying KL, Seeger RC. Deletion of chromosome 11 and of 14q sequences in neuroblastoma. *Genes Chromosomes Cancer* 1993;7:32–7.
14. Janoueix-Lerosey I, Schleiermacher G, Michels E et al. Overall genomic pattern is a predictor of outcome in neuroblastoma. *J Clin Oncol* 2009;27:1026–33.
15. Pinto N, Naranjo A, Hibbitts E et al. Predictors of differential response to induction therapy in high-risk neuroblastoma: a report from the Children's Oncology Group (COG). *Eur J Cancer* 2019;112:66–79.

16. Irwin MS, Naranjo A, Zhang FF et al. Revised neuroblastoma risk classification system: a report from the Children's Oncology Group. *J Clin Oncol* 2021;39:3229–41.
17. Sokol E, Desai AV, Applebaum MA et al. Age, diagnostic category, tumor grade, and mitosis-karyorrhexis index are independently prognostic in neuroblastoma: an INRG project. *J Clin Oncol* 2020;38:1906–18.
18. Moreno L, Caron H, Geoerger B et al. Accelerating drug development for neuroblastoma – New Drug Development Strategy: an Innovative Therapies for Children with Cancer, European Network for Cancer Research in Children and Adolescents and International Society of Paediatric Oncology Europe Neuroblastoma project. *Expert Opin Drug Discov* 2017; 12:801–11.
19. Pugh TJ, Morozova O, Attiyeh EF et al. The genetic landscape of high-risk neuroblastoma. *Nat Genet* 2013;45:279–84.
20. Je EM, Choi YJ, Yoo NJ, Lee SH. Oncogenic PTPN11 mutations are rare in solid tumors. *Pathol Oncol Res* 2015;21:225–7.

3 Diagnosis

Oncology

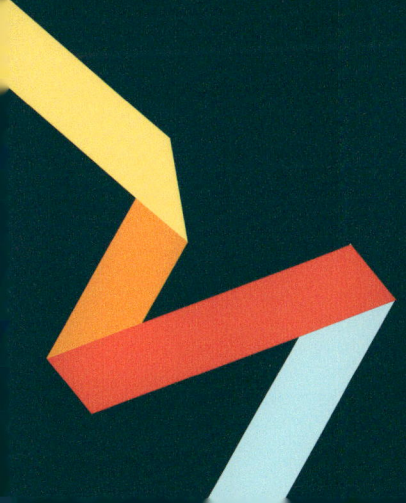

HEALTHCARE

Clinical presentation

Neuroblastoma is the most common extracranial solid-tumor malignancy in childhood. Most cases occur in children aged under 5 years, although it can occur in adolescence and adulthood. Neuroblastoma may arise from the adrenal gland or anywhere else along the sympathetic chain. The most common primary site of disease is within the abdomen (adrenal [47%], retroperitoneal [24%]), followed by the mediastinum (thoracic sympathetic ganglia [15%]), cervical sympathetic ganglia (3%) and, lastly, the pelvic sympathetic ganglia (3%).[1]

Presenting symptoms based on primary tumor location

Intra-abdominal masses can lead to children presenting with constipation, abdominal pain or distension, and fussiness. Physical examination may identify a fixed abdominal mass that crosses the midline with borders that are difficult to appreciate because of its site of origin. Large intra-abdominal masses can result in abdominal compartment syndrome and respiratory distress.[2]

Masses within the mediastinum and neck, along the thoracic or cervical sympathetic chain, may be found incidentally without other associated symptoms. However, children may present with Horner syndrome (unilateral ptosis, miosis and anhidrosis). Large tumors in this area can also result in airway compression or superior vena cava syndrome.[2]

Paraspinal tumors that invade the neural foramina of adjacent vertebral bodies can cause neurological symptoms such as numbness, weakness, bladder and/or bowel dysfunction, and radicular pain. This is considered a medical emergency and should be managed as such (see page 56).[2]

Constitutional symptoms that patients may present with include:
- fatigue
- loss of appetite
- weight loss
- pallor
- elevated blood pressure.

Other symptoms may result from disease metastasis. Neuroblastoma can spread through the lymphatic system as well as by hematogenous dissemination. Common sites of metastasis are listed in Table 3.1.

Paraneoplastic syndromes either result from abnormal chemokine secretion by the tumor or an abnormal host immune response to the malignant cells in which immune cells start attacking the normal host cells in addition to cancerous cells. There are two syndromes associated with neuroblastoma.

Opsoclonus-myoclonus-ataxia syndrome (OMAS) is observed in 2–3% of newly diagnosed patients with neuroblastoma, and is associated with localized disease and favorable prognosis. However, 70–80% of patients continue to have long-term neurological deficits such as cognitive delay, motor delay, language deficits and abnormal behaviors. This is presumed to be secondary to neural antibodies,

TABLE 3.1

Common sites of metastasis[2]

Site	Description
Lymph nodes	Patients may have regional as well as distant lymph node metastases
Bone marrow and cortical bone	Can result in bone pain and limp; laboratory examination often shows cytopenias in patients with bone marrow metastases
Periorbital bones	Can cause periorbital ecchymosis, resulting in characteristic 'raccoon eyes' (Figure 3.1)
Liver	Patients may present with abdominal pain and distension with hepatomegaly on physical examination
Skin	Appear as diffusely distributed, non-tender, bluish subcutaneous nodules, most commonly in infants, resulting in 'blueberry muffin' appearance (Figure 3.2)
Lungs and CNS	Rare; when it does occur, it is usually in relapsing or end-stage disease

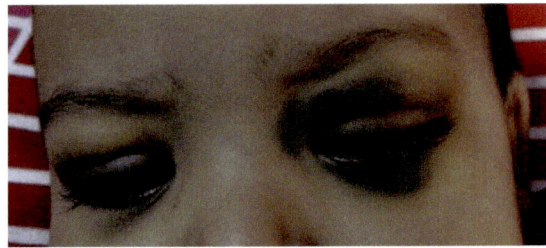

Figure 3.1 'Raccoon eyes' caused by periorbital ecchymosis. Reproduced with permission from Kapoor and Chabbra 2014.[3]

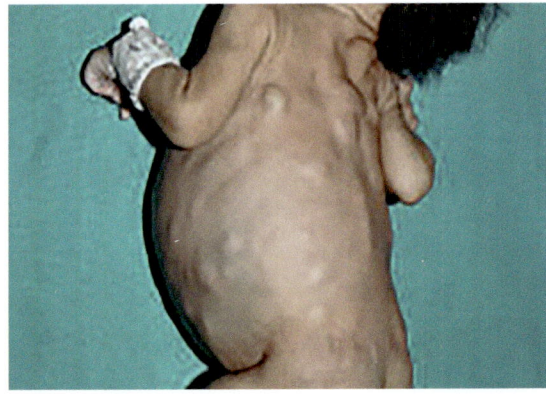

Figure 3.2 Multiple light bluish subcutaneous nodules over the trunk cause the 'blueberry muffin' appearance characteristic of neuroblastoma. Reproduced with permission from Kumar et al. 2018.[4]

formed against the tumor, that persist and cross-react with normal neural cells.

OMAS is characterized by:
- abnormal eye movements
- episodes of jerky, spastic movements
- ataxia or uncoordinated movements.

Symptoms may wax and wane, with exacerbation noted during intercurrent infections. Children who present with OMAS should undergo workup for neuroblastoma including full-body MRI and possibly scintigraphy with ^{123}I-meta-iodobenzylguanidine (^{123}I-MIBG) (see pages 36–7). Treatment for OMAS includes intravenous immunoglobulin, chemotherapy, glucocorticoids, and rituximab and/or other immunosuppressive agents for which there are ongoing clinical trials.[2]

Vasoactive intestinal peptide syndrome is due to vasoactive intestinal peptide (VIP) secretion by the tumor and is characterized by:
- intractable watery diarrhea with abdominal distension
- resultant hypokalemia
- dehydration.

Tumors that are associated with VIP syndrome are often histologically mature (such as ganglioneuroblastoma or ganglioneuroma). Patients with such tumors have favorable prognoses. Symptoms associated with VIP syndrome usually resolve after tumor resection.[2]

Diagnosis

Based on international consensus, a diagnosis of neuroblastoma is established by either of the following criteria.[5]
- Tumor histology by light microscopy, with or without immunohistology (see Light microscopy, pages 33–4).
- Bone marrow aspirate or biopsy findings consistent with metastatic disease, in addition to elevated urinary catecholamine metabolite levels (see Initial analysis, pages 32–3).

Perinatal diagnosis. Most prenatally detected cases of neuroblastoma are of adrenal origin and are usually detected during the third trimester. Tumors can present as a solid mass with or without cystic features and/or calcification on ultrasound. Fetal MRI may be helpful to obtain more information regarding tumor size, position and invasion into nearby structures. Differential diagnoses that may be considered include:
- adrenal hemorrhage
- congenital adrenal hyperplasia
- pulmonary sequestration
- renal duplication
- splenic or hepatic cyst.

Postnatal diagnosis. Infants should undergo ultrasonography to confirm the presence of an adrenal mass and subsequent advanced imaging, by either CT or MRI, is obtained as further workup. If there is continued concern for neonatal neuroblastoma, complete workup with laboratory evaluation and ^{123}I-MIBG scintigraphy (see pages 36–7) is conducted.[6–8] Differential diagnoses in pediatric patients include:
- Wilms tumor, hepatoblastoma, renal cell carcinoma and congenital mesoblastic nephroma for intra-abdominal tumors
- lymphoma, rhabdomyosarcoma and extraosseous Ewing sarcoma for mediastinal/cervical masses
- ganglioneuroma and ganglioneuroblastoma for tumors that arise from the sympathetic ganglia
- other CNS tumors such as astrocytomas, epidermoid tumors, desmoid tumors and teratomas for tumors that involve the spine[9]
- other infiltrative diseases such as leukemia for disease involving the bone marrow.

History taking and physical examination should be thoroughly undertaken for all patients with suspected neuroblastoma. Physical examination findings may be non-specific and depend on the location of the tumor (see page 28). Careful abdominal examination to palpate for an abdominal mass and assessment of hepatomegaly and lymphadenopathy is required.

Laboratory evaluation
Initial analysis includes complete blood count (CBC), coagulation studies, serum chemistries and liver panel analysis. Lactate dehydrogenase and serum ferritin levels may also be assessed. If CBCs indicate cytopenias, especially if there is metastasis to the bone marrow, patients may require transfusions at diagnosis depending on the severity of anemia and thrombocytopenia. Additional laboratory findings that may be notable include elevated erythrocyte sedimentation rate and serum ferritin levels, as well as elevated transaminases on a liver panel. Rarely, neuroblastoma can cause 'syndrome of inappropriate antidiuretic hormone secretion', which results in hyponatremia; however, this is more common in adult patients.

Because of their noradrenergic origins, neuroblastomas often express the enzymes monoamine oxidase and catechol-*O*-methyltransferase, which are involved in catecholamine synthesis. As a result, 70–80% of patients with neuroblastoma have elevated serum and urine levels of the catecholamine metabolites homovanillic acid and vanillylmandelic acid. If elevated, these urine markers are useful in aiding diagnosis.[2]

Virtual karyotyping can be performed on fresh or paraffin-embedded tissue to assess copy number at the locus of interest. For neuroblastoma tumor samples, array-based copy number analysis is feasible, although single-nucleotide polymorphism (SNP) array virtual karyotyping is preferred because this can detect copy-neutral LOH (for example, acquired uniparental disomy where both gene copies originate from the same parental chromosome, which can be effectively equivalent to a deletion). SNP array virtual karyotyping can detect LOH such as is seen with 1p or 11p deletion, as well as detecting MYC-N amplification and 17q gain.[10] However, standard array comparative genomic hybridization, FISH and conventional cytogenetics cannot detect copy-neutral LOH.

Light microscopy. Biopsy samples should be obtained by an experienced surgeon after consultation with an oncologist. It is important that adequate tissue is obtained during biopsy sampling to enable complete characterization of the tumor. Diagnostic tissue is often obtained by incisional or image-guided core needle biopsy.

When viewed by light microscopy, neuroblastoma tumors are characterized by 'small round blue cells' that are uniformly sized, containing dense, hyperchromatic nuclei with scant cytoplasm. A characteristic feature of neuroblastoma cells is the presence of neuritic processes called neuropils. A classic, but infrequent, finding on histology is the Homer Wright pseudorosette, which is a central core of eosinophilic neuropils surrounded by a ring of neuroblasts (Figure 3.3). Evaluation of stromal presence, degree of neural differentiation and mitosis-karyorrhexis index determines whether the tumor presents with favorable or unfavorable histology.

While other neoplasms, such as Ewing sarcoma and rhabdomyosarcoma, are associated with 'small round blue cells', experienced pathologists are usually able to distinguish between them and neuroblastoma. Immunohistochemical stains (Table 3.2)

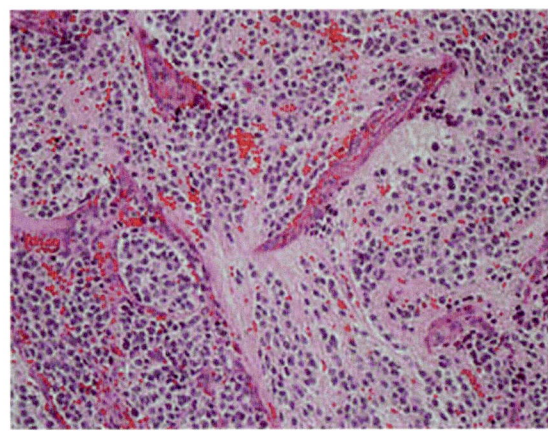

Figure 3.3 Poorly differentiated neuroblastoma, with nests of neuroblasts in a background of light pink fibrillary neuropil (magnification ×100). Reproduced with permission from Pizzo and Poplack 1993.[11]

TABLE 3.2

Immunohistochemical staining results for neuroblastoma cells[2]

Positive	Negative
Neuron-specific antibodies against tyrosine hydroxylase, neuron-specific enolase, synaptophysin, chromogranin, CD56, CD57, protein gene product 9.5, Leu-7, disialoganglioside GD2, NB84, neurofilament protein, ALK (>90% stain positively), PHOX2B, glial fibrillary acidic protein	Epithelial membrane antigen, cytokeratin, vimentin, HMB45, Wilms tumor protein, CD99, CD45, desmin, myogenin, myoblast determination protein 1, S100

and molecular testing methods are available that can be helpful in establishing pathological diagnosis.[2]

Imaging

Radiographs can have a non-specific appearance, revealing a soft tissue mass. Skeletal metastases detected on radiographs are often described as ill-defined and lucent. Periosteal reaction or metaphysical lucency may be reported.

Ultrasound imaging of neuroblastomas often observes them to be heterogeneous with internal vascularity. There may be areas of low echogenicity that may represent tumor necrosis.

CT scanning enables the visualization of more detailed findings associated with the primary tumor. Again, masses are typically heterogeneous, with 80–90% of cases revealing calcification within the tumor. CT findings of the primary tumor and its mass effect on the surrounding organs, vessels and vertebral body will depend on the size, location and aggressive nature of the primary tumor (Figure 3.4). Lymph node enlargement is a common finding.[12]

MRI is superior to other modalities in obtaining details regarding the organ of origin, lymphadenopathy, invasion into adjacent structures or vessels, and intracranial or intraspinal disease, as well as bone marrow involvement. T1 imaging will reveal a heterogeneous mass that is iso- to hypointense, similar to that seen on

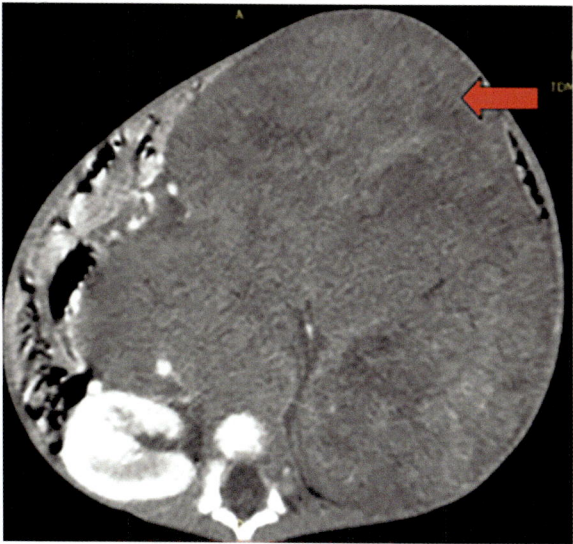

Figure 3.4 Abdominal pelvic CT scan shows a large retroperitoneal tissue mass crossing the midline (arrow) in a 3-year-old girl. Reproduced with permission under the terms of the Creative Commons Attribution License from Yessoufou-Bakary et al. 2015.[13]

ultrasonography or CT imaging. On T2 imaging, the heterogeneity is characterized by hyperintense areas that are reflective of cystic or necrotic areas of the tumor.[14]

Staging workup

It is imperative that staging studies are completed prior to initiating therapy. The goal of these studies is to evaluate the extent of disease, which in turn plays an important role in risk stratification and subsequent treatment. These evaluations are best completed at a pediatric cancer center where experienced oncologists and radiologists can be closely involved in the coordination and planning of studies.

Imaging of the primary tumor and suspected sites of metastasis should comprise either CT or MRI. Upon confirmation of the diagnosis, patients with neuroblastoma should be evaluated for metastatic disease by scintigraphy with ^{123}I-MIBG. MIBG is an analog of norepinephrine, which specifically allows for uptake by neuroendocrine cells. By tagging MIBG with radioactive iodine, active areas of disease can be detected by scintigraphy (Figure 3.5). MIBG uptake by cortical bone is never normal and should raise concern of metastatic disease. ^{123}I-MIBG scans are assessed using the Curie scoring system, which divides the skeleton into nine segments, with an additional tenth segment for soft tissue disease. Each segment receives a score of 0–3 depending on the extent of disease (Tables 3.3 and 3.4).[15]

A small percentage of patients have non-avid disease on ^{123}I-MIBG scintigraphy and should alternatively be evaluated with fluorodeoxyglucose-positron emission tomography to detect metastasis to cortical bone.

The last component in staging workup for neuroblastoma is analysis of bone marrow aspirates and biopsy samples. Samples should be obtained from two separate sites, usually bilateral iliac crests. Four samples (two aspirates and two biopsy samples) should be evaluated for the presence of tumor cells and all four must be without evidence of malignancy to be considered negative.

Diagnosis

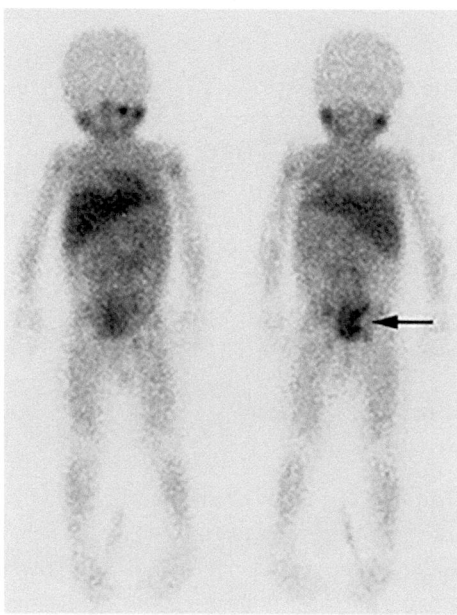

Figure 3.5 ¹²³I-MIBG scan images of a 2-year-old boy with metastatic neuroblastoma. Anterior (left) and posterior (right) whole-body ¹²³I-MIBG planar images obtained with a bladder catheter in place show ¹²³I-MIBG uptake in an irregular pelvic mass, which is more intense on the posterior image (arrow). Abnormal ¹²³I-MIBG uptake is also seen in sites of skeletal metastatic disease, most notably involving the face, proximal humeri, spine and pelvis. Reproduced with permission from Sharp et al. 2016.[15]

TABLE 3.3

Curie skeleton scoring system

Curie score	Extent of disease
0	No disease
1	Single site of disease
2	2+ sites of disease, with <50% involvement of segment
3	2+ sites of disease, with >50% involvement of segment

TABLE 3.4

Curie soft tissue scoring system

Curie score	Extent of disease
0	No disease
1	Single site of disease (soft tissue)
2	2+ sites of disease (soft tissue)
3	Soft tissue lesion occupying >50% of chest or abdomen

 Key points – diagnosis

- Diagnosis of neuroblastoma is established by either of the following criteria: (a) tumor histology by light microscopy, with or without immunohistology, or (b) bone marrow aspirate or biopsy findings consistent with metastatic disease, in addition to elevated urinary catecholamine metabolite levels.
- Neuroblastoma can present in a variety of ways depending on location. The most common site of primary disease is intra-abdominal.
- There are two associated paraneoplastic syndromes, OMAS and VIP syndrome. OMAS is characterized by abnormal eye movements as well as spasmodic body movements. This is secondary to an immune response against the neuroblastoma tumor. VIP syndrome is characterized by intractable watery diarrhea caused by VIP secretion by tumor cells.
- Under light microscopy, neuroblastoma tumors are characterized by 'small round blue cells'. A characteristic feature of neuroblastoma cells is the presence of neuritic processes called neuropils.
- It is imperative that staging workup for neuroblastoma is completed before the initiation of therapy, with a few clinical exceptions due to clinical status.

References

1. Vo KT, Matthay KK, Neuhaus J et al. Clinical, biologic, and prognostic differences on the basis of primary tumor site in neuroblastoma: a report from the international neuroblastoma risk group project. *J Clin Oncol* 2014;32:3169–76.
2. Brodeur G, Hogarty M, Bagatell R et al. Neuroblastoma. In: Pizzo PA, Poplack DG, eds. *Principles and Practice of Pediatric Oncology*, 7th edn. Wolters Kluwer; 2016.
3. Kapoor PG, Chabbra R. Neuroblastoma presenting as raccoon eyes. *J Pediatr* 2014;164:1495.
4. Kumar M, Batra G, Saun A et al. Blueberry muffin baby: an unusual presentation of infantile neuroblastoma. *Indian J Med Paediatr Oncol* 2018;39:263–5.
5. Brodeur GM, Pritchard J, Berthold F et al. Revisions of the international criteria for neuroblastoma diagnosis, staging, and response to treatment. *J Clin Oncol* 1993;11:1466–77.
6. Davidoff A. Neonatal neuroblastoma. *Clin Perinatol* 2021;48:101–115.
7. Lesieur E, Noire A, Maurice P et al. Prenatal assessment of atypical adrenal glands. *J Ultrasound Med* 2021;40:1719–28.
8. Psarris A, Sindos M, Dimopoulou A et al. Prenatal diagnosis of adrenal neuroblastoma – differential diagnosis of suprarenal masses in the third trimester of pregnancy. *Ultrasound Int Open* 2019;5:E93–5.
9. Wilson RE, Oleszek JL, Clayton GH. Pediatric spinal cord tumors and masses. *J Spinal Cord Med* 2007;30:S15–20.
10. Carén H, Erichsen J, Olsson L et al. High-resolution array copy number analyses for detection of deletion, gain, amplification and copy-neutral LOH in primary neuroblastoma tumors: four cases of homozygous deletions of the CDKN2A gene. *BMC Genomics* 2008;9:353.
11. Pizzo PA, Poplack DG. *Principles and Practice of Pediatric Oncology*, 2nd edn. J.B. Lippincott, 1993.
12. Kembhavi SA, Shah S, Rangarajan V et al. Imaging in neuroblastoma: an update. *Indian J Radiol Imaging* 2015;25:129–36.
13. Yessoufou-Bakary N, Kouamé N, Manewa S et al. Neuroblastoma: radiological diagnosis of a case with pulmonary metastases. *Int J Radiol Imaging Technol* 2015;1:007.
14. Dumba M, Jawad N, McHugh K. Neuroblastoma and nephroblastoma: a radiological review. *Cancer Imaging* 2015;15:5.
15. Sharp SE, Trout AT, Weiss BD, Gelfand MJ. MIBG in neuroblastoma diagnostic imaging and therapy. *Radiographics* 2016;36:258–78.

4 Staging and risk stratification

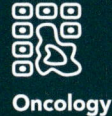
Oncology

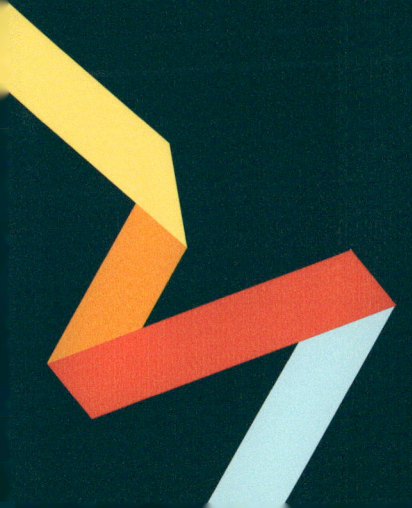

HEALTHCARE

Staging systems

The International Neuroblastoma Staging System (INSS) was adopted in the 1990s and was the first staging system to provide uniformity among clinical trials and biological studies worldwide. Disease staging is based on tumor resection and spread to lymph nodes, as well as other metastatic sites (Table 4.1).[1]

The International Neuroblastoma Risk Group Staging System (INRGSS) was developed in 2009 as a revised version of the INSS. This staging system is based on clinical features (Table 4.2), incorporates

TABLE 4.1

Stages in the INSS

Stage	Description
1	Localized tumor with GTR, with or without microscopic residual disease; ipsilateral lymph nodes obtained for sampling must be negative for tumor microscopically, but lymph nodes attached to and removed with the primary tumor may be positive
2A	Localized tumor with incomplete GTR; representative ipsilateral non-adherent lymph nodes are negative microscopically
2B	Localized tumor with or without GTR, with positive ipsilateral non-adherent lymph nodes; contralateral lymph nodes that are enlarged must be sampled and negative microscopically
3	Unresectable unilateral tumor that crosses the midline, with or without regional lymph node involvement OR Localized unilateral tumor with contralateral regional lymph node involvement OR Midline tumor with bilateral extension either by tumor infiltration or lymph node involvement
4	Any primary tumor with spread to distant lymph nodes, bone, bone marrow, liver, skin and/or other organs
4S	Applicable only to patients aged < 1 year, with localized primary tumor (as defined by stage 1, 2A or 2B), with metastatic sites limited to skin, liver and/or bone marrow

GTR, gross total resection.

TABLE 4.2

Stages in the INRGSS

Stage	Description
L1	Localized tumor, confined to one body compartment, without involvement of vital structures as defined by list of IDRFs
L2	Locoregional tumor with one or more IDRFs
M	Distant metastatic disease (excluding stage MS)
MS	Metastatic disease confined to skin, liver and/or bone marrow in children aged < 18 months

IDRF, image-defined risk factor.

imaging parameters at diagnosis (Table 4.3) and does not rely on the extent of surgical excision. Data suggest that the INRGSS provides improved insight into which patients require more intensive treatment and it is now used by all international cooperative groups, including the COG.[2,3]

Prognosis and risk stratification

The International Neuroblastoma Risk Group risk-classification system. Patient prognosis and treatment are based on the International Neuroblastoma Risk Group (INRG) risk-classification system. This system takes into account the patient's age at diagnosis, INRGSS stage, primary tumor site, histology, ploidy, presence of *MYCN* amplification and SCAs (Figure 4.1).[4]

INRG stage L1. Patients with L1 tumors aged under 12 months with maximum tumor diameters less than 5 cm are considered to have favorable features. These patients are eligible to be observed with watchful waiting on the current non-high-risk COG protocol ANBL1232. Patients aged under 12 months with L1 tumors larger than 5 cm at maximum diameter may be observed after gross total resection (GTR); however, patients who undergo incomplete resection will be treated according to their *MYCN* status. Patients whose tumors are negative for *MYCN* amplification are considered low risk and may be observed; however, those with *MYCN* amplification are stratified into the high-risk group.

TABLE 4.3

Image-defined risk factors on the INRGSS

Tumor location	Description
General	• Ipsilateral tumor extension within two body compartments (i.e. neck–chest, chest–abdomen, abdomen–pelvis)
	• Infiltration of pericardium, diaphragm, kidney, liver, duodenopancreatic block, mesentery
Neck	• Tumor encasement of carotid and/or vertebral artery and/or internal jugular vein
	• Tumor extension to base of skull
	• Tracheal compression
Cervicothoracic	• Tumor encasement of brachial plexus roots
	• Tumor encasement of subclavian vessels and/or vertebral artery and/or carotid artery
	• Tracheal compression
Thorax	• Tumor encasement of aorta and/or major branches
	• Tracheal compression or compression of principal bronchi
	• Infiltration of costovertebral junction between T9 and T12
Thoracoabdominal	• Tumor encasement of the aorta and/or vena cava
Abdomen/pelvis	• Tumor infiltration of porta hepatis and/or hepatoduodenal ligament
	• Tumor encasement of the branches of the superior mesenteric artery at the mesenteric root
	• Tumor encasement of the origin of the celiac axis and/or of the superior mesenteric artery
	• Tumor invasion to one or both renal pedicles
	• Tumor encasement of the aorta and/or vena cava
	• Tumor encasement of the iliac vessels
	• Pelvic tumor crossing the sciatic notch
Intraspinal	• Invasion into more than one-third of the spinal canal in the axial plane
	• Loss of visibility of the perimedullary leptomeningeal spaces
	• Abnormal spinal cord signal

Patients with L1 tumors who are aged 12 months or older who undergo GTR of their tumor are considered low risk and can be observed after surgery; however, for those with incomplete resection, risk stratification depends on *MYCN* amplification. Patients without amplification can be observed, while those with *MYCN* amplification are treated as high risk.

INRG stage L2. Patients with L2 tumors with *MYCN* amplification, regardless of age, histology and biomarkers, are considered high risk and treated as such. In rare clinical situations, L2 *MYCN*-amplified tumors may have been fully resected and could potentially be closely observed, though the risk of relapse is high. Patients aged under 18 months without *MYCN* amplification, regardless of histology or cytogenetics, are considered intermediate risk. Those between the ages of 18 months and 5 years without *MYCN* amplification and with favorable histology are stratified as intermediate risk, while those with unfavorable histology are considered high risk. Risk stratification for patients without *MYCN* amplification but aged 5 years or older depends on the degree of differentiation by histology. Those with differentiating tumors are intermediate risk, while those with undifferentiated or poorly differentiated tumors are high risk.

INRG stage M. Patients with metastatic disease (stage M) aged under 12 months are considered intermediate risk if there is no *MYCN* amplification. If the patient is between 12 and 18 months of age without *MYCN* amplification, risk stratification depends on biomarkers. Those with favorable histology, no SCAs and with ploidy greater than 1 are stratified into the intermediate-risk group; however, if biomarkers are unfavorable (unfavorable histology, diploid or with SCAs) then patients are considered high risk. Patients at any age with *MYCN* amplification and those older than 18 months of age regardless of *MYCN* amplification status are considered high risk.

INRG stage MS. Patients younger than 12 months of age with INRG stage MS disease without *MYCN* amplification or tumor-related symptoms, but with favorable biomarkers, are considered low risk. If biomarkers are unfavorable, these patients are considered intermediate risk. Infant patients (<12 months of age) with tumor-related symptoms such as respiratory distress, hepatitis, renal insufficiency and coagulopathy are also considered intermediate risk.

(a)

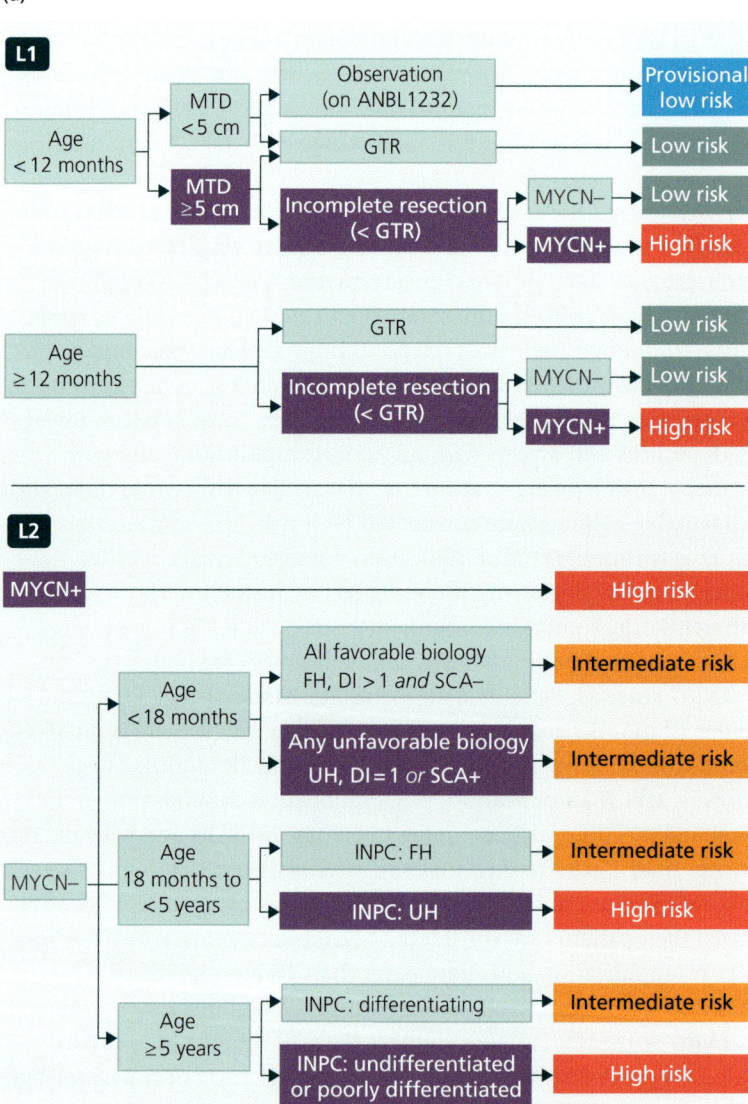

Figure 4.1 INRGSS risk classifier version 2 algorithm for patients with locoregional and metastatic tumors. (a) Patients with locoregional tumors with neuroblastoma and ganglioneuroblastoma (nodular) are classified based on INRG stage (L1 and L2), age, resection, biomarkers (*MYCN* status, ploidy and SCAs) and INPC.

(b)

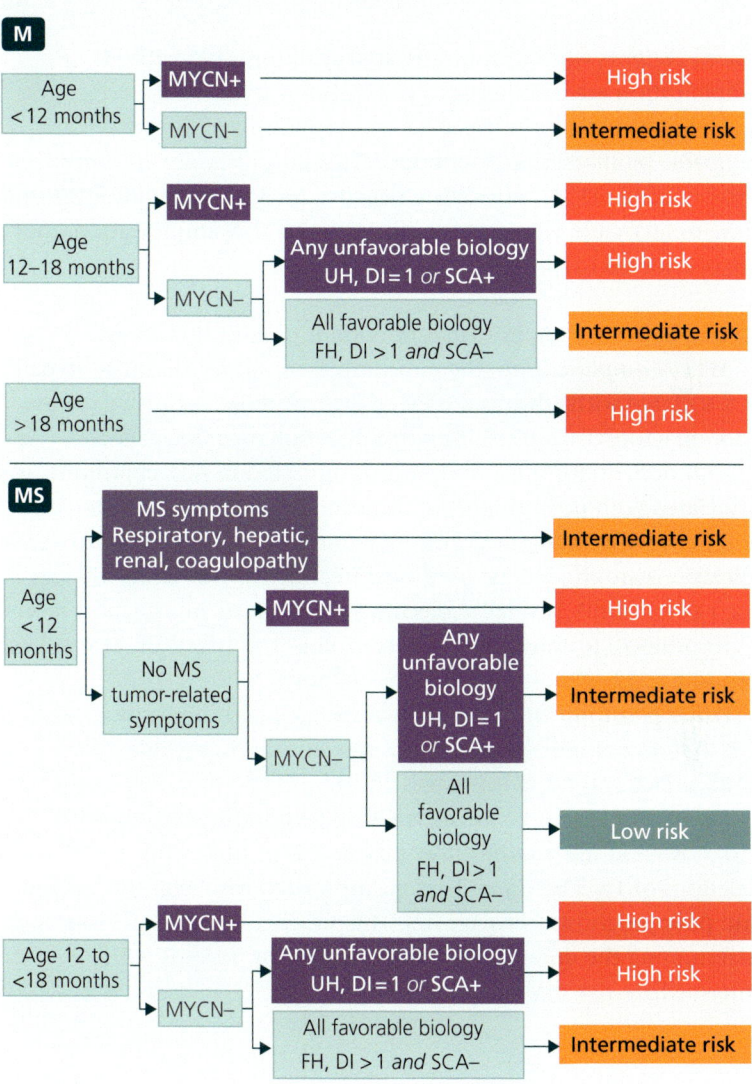

Figure 4.1 *(CONTD)* (b) Patients with metastatic tumors are classified by stage (M and MS), age, INPC and biomarkers. DI, DNA index; FH, favorable histology; INPC, International Neuroblastoma Pathology Classifier; MTD, maximum tumor diameter; MYCN+, *MYCN* amplified; MYCN–, *MYCN* not amplified; UH, unfavorable histology. Reproduced with permission from Irwin et al. 2021.[4]

Infant patients without tumor-related symptoms but with *MYCN* amplification are stratified into the high-risk group.

Similarly, patients between 12 and 18 months of age with favorable biomarkers and without *MYCN* amplification are considered intermediate risk. If patients are negative for *MYCN* amplification and have unfavorable biomarkers or they have *MYCN* amplification, they are considered to have high-risk disease.

Cytogenetics are implicated as important prognostic factors.

MYCN amplification, the most important factor identified to date, is associated with advanced stage of disease, more aggressive disease and refractory disease resulting in a poor outcome (see page 22).

ALK activation, the most frequent mutation in neuroblastoma, is associated with poor prognosis; however, it is potentially targetable, and patients with high-risk disease found to have ALK-activating gene alterations are eligible for additional treatment with ALK inhibitors such as crizotinib, a small-molecule ALK inhibitor, on the most recent COG protocol for high-risk neuroblastoma. The effects on EFS and OS of adding ALK inhibition are as yet unknown.[5]

Other point mutations that are associated with high-risk disease but that do not yet play a role in risk stratification include *PTPN11*, *TERT*, *ATRX* and *NRAS* (see pages 22–4).

Segmental chromosome aberrations play an important role in prognosis and risk stratification. Gains of 17q, 1q and 2p, as well as deletions of 1p, 11q, 3p and 4p, are associated with aggressive disease and poor prognosis (see page 22). The presence of SCAs plays a role in determining the duration of chemotherapy for patients with intermediate-risk disease.

Key points – staging and risk stratification

- The INSS is based on tumor resection and spread to lymph nodes, as well as other metastatic sites, and has been retired in favor of the INRGSS.
- The INRGSS is based on clinical features and incorporates imaging parameters at diagnosis.
- The INRGSS is now used by all international cooperative groups, such as the COG.
- Important prognostic factors include INRG staging, age at diagnosis, the presence or absence of *MYCN* amplification, histology, and biomarkers such as diploidy and SCAs.
- The most important prognostic cytogenetic finding in neuroblastoma tumor cells is *MYCN* amplification.

References

1. Brodeur GM, Pritchard J, Berthold F et al. Revisions of the international criteria for neuroblastoma diagnosis, staging, and response to treatment. *J Clin Oncol* 1993;11:1466–77.
2. Monclair T, Brodeur GM, Ambros PF et al. The International Neuroblastoma Risk Group (INRG) Staging System: an INRG Task Force report. *J Clin Oncol* 2009;27:298–303.
3. Cohn SL, Pearson ADJ, London WB et al. The International Neuroblastoma Risk Group (INRG) classification system: an INRG Task Force report. *J Clin Oncol* 2009;27:289–97.
4. Irwin MS, Naranjo A, Zhang FF et al. Revised neuroblastoma risk classification system: a report from the Children's Oncology Group. *J Clin Oncol* 2021;39:3229–41.
5. Bellini A, Pötschger U, Bernard V et al. Frequency and prognostic impact of *ALK* amplifications and mutations in the European Neuroblastoma Study Group (SIOPEN) High-Risk Neuroblastoma Trial (HR-NBL1). *J Clin Oncol* 2021;39:3377–90.

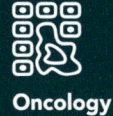

5 Management

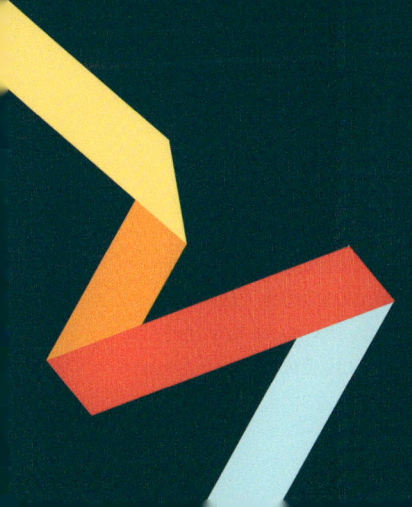

HEALTHCARE

Just as there is a wide range of clinical presentations for neuroblastoma, treatment also varies from watching and waiting to integrated multimodal treatment with chemotherapy, surgical resection, bone marrow transplantation, radiotherapy and immunotherapy. The development of current treatment regimens has resulted from multicenter clinical trials run by cooperative groups such as the COG in the USA and the International Society of Paediatric Oncology European Neuroblastoma Group (SIOPEN) in Europe.

Surgery

Surgical decisions are a critical component of the multimodal treatment plan and guide clinical pathways from the mechanisms of biopsy, central venous access for chemotherapy administration and definitive local control tumor resection. In the USA, the current standard surgical treatments for neuroblastoma are guided by protocols established by COG clinical trials. The critical surgical goals are to establish diagnosis, determine accurate staging, and conduct the most complete surgical resection that preserves organ function and avoids disability.

Surgical standards

For patients with low-risk tumors, surgical standards revolve around establishing diagnosis and achieving maximal surgical resection with preservation of surrounding organs and function. This approach is based on the results of COG study P9641, which demonstrated 3-year OS of at least 95% in asymptomatic low-risk patients with stage 1, 2a and 2b neuroblastomas after surgery alone.[1] The goals are to minimize surgical risks and limit chemotherapy in patients with favorable biological features. The general surgical principals for patients in this risk group are to resect as much tumor as safely possible without damage to contiguous structures or major blood vessels. For resectability, surgeons utilize the INRG image-defined risk factors (IDRFs) to assess if resection can be achieved upfront.

Tumors in this risk group are typically L1 tumors and are safely resected without surgical complications. Neuroblastoma tumors may be found in the neck, chest, abdomen and pelvis, and tend to cluster at the sympathetic neuronal chain, adrenal gland, organ of Zuckerkandl and on major blood vessels without invasion beyond the tunica adventitia. Chemotherapy in this group is reserved for patients with less than 50% resection or relapsed disease, and radiotherapy is seldom given.

Stage MS neuroblastoma tumors may be spared both surgery and chemotherapy. This subset of tumors often spontaneously regress, but exceptions are patients with massive hepatomegaly from liver metastases causing intra-abdominal hypertension and abdominal compartment syndrome. In such situations, patients may require decompressive laparotomy and ventilator support. For these reasons, patients with a large liver tumor burden require extra-abdominal sites for biopsy to establish the diagnosis. In such cases, treatment via chemotherapy may be initiated to decrease the intra-abdominal tumor burden.

For patients with intermediate-risk tumors, as for low-risk tumors, the priority is to establish the diagnosis and achieve complete resection without compromising organ function. The surgeon should utilize INRG IDRFs to assess resectability.

For intermediate-risk tumors with L2 characteristics, biopsy is performed with planning for neoadjuvant chemotherapy. It is critical to obtain enough tissue for histological and genetic analysis because the biology of the tumor will drive the treatment plan. Delayed surgical resection, if needed, is then typically completed after 4–6 cycles of chemotherapy. The goals of care of children in this risk group center upon reducing cytotoxic therapy and surgical resection.

For patients with high-risk tumors, surgical resection is typically performed at the same time as induction chemotherapy (see pages 60–1), and surgical standards are the most challenging. Survival rates in this group remain poor despite multimodal therapy, and initial management begins with adequate operative or percutaneous biopsy and venous access placement. The surgeon should obtain at least 1–2 cm^3 of tumor tissue for histopathological analysis. Core needle biopsies may be utilized with attention to detail around obtaining high-volume viable specimens from adequate core numbers, and perioperative pathological assessment for adequacy.[2] The quality of the biopsy specimen, open or percutaneous, should be confirmed with the pathologist prior to leaving the operating room. Most patients in this group will have high response rates to chemotherapy and improved tumor resectability. Local control is achieved with a combination of surgical resection and external-beam radiotherapy to the primary tumor site. The role of primary total tumor resection in this group of patients has been controversial, with the most recent studies in the USA and abroad showing that removal of more than 90% of the primary tumor improves survival and decreases local recurrence.[3]

Gross total resection is defined as the clearing of all visible and palpable tumor from the primary tumor bed and regional lymph node tissue. Under the INRGSS, lymph node dissection is not required, although any nodes that appear abnormal should be excised. The goals are to achieve GTR, keeping in mind that the microscopic margins are nearly always positive. In most cases, safe dissection begins by exposing the involved great vessels and spine, and systematically clearing the tumor from all involved spaces with meticulous dissection in the peritumoral capsular plane. Safe surgical techniques are utilized in tumor resections in the neck, thorax, and abdomen or pelvis. In patients with high-risk neuroblastoma, GTR typically takes place after cycle 4 of induction chemotherapy.

Thoracic neuroblastomas are characterized by generally more favorable biology and better survival rates than abdominal and pelvic tumors, and surgical resection is often curative. Tumors less than 6 cm in size may be safely approached thoracoscopically to avoid open thoracotomy.[4,5] Tumors at the cervical chain may present challenges around the great vessels and the trachea, and a radical neck incision may be required. Effort should be made to avoid injury to the vagus and phrenic nerves. For tumors that extend beyond the thoracic inlet into the chest, a trapdoor incision may be utilized to safely approach the tumor and achieve total resection.

Abdominal and pelvic neuroblastomas may encroach upon renal vessels and the kidney. Tumors less than 6 cm in size that are limited to the adrenal gland may be approached laparoscopically. For open operations, the incision type depends upon the location of the primary tumor and thoracoabdominal incisions may be beneficial for large masses that approach the diaphragm and crus. Meticulous effort should be made to avoid renal injury or nephrectomy, particularly in patients with high-risk tumors who will need adequate renal function to tolerate cytotoxic therapy and myeloablative agents. Tumors may involve the aorta, vena cava, celiac axis, superior mesenteric artery and inferior mesenteric artery, and are often tightly adherent, although not typically invasive beyond the adventitia. Given this, it is beneficial to divide the tumor over major blood vessels and obtain safe exposure for removal when en-bloc resection is not possible because of encased blood vessels. The lumbosacral plexus should be avoided and innervation to the bladder and reproductive organs should be preserved. For tumors that involve the pelvic sidewall, intraoperative nerve stimulation and monitoring may be useful. MRI to determine the extent of spinal involvement may help surgical planning.

Operative complications are site dependent. Early control of the aorta and vena cava provides the safest operative technique to trace major vessels and provide complete GTR. All efforts should be made to avoid nephrectomy, bowel resection, or lymphatic and nerve injuries. Such complications may also slow the recovery phase and delay chemotherapy and radiotherapy. Tightly adherent areas should be left rather than risk injury. Other complications such as chylous leak, infection and abscess are rare, and should be handled promptly to expedite healing and the completion of ongoing therapy.

Radiotherapy

Radiotherapy is a mainstay of local regional control for patients with high-risk neuroblastoma and some patients with intermediate-risk disease. Radiotherapy typically occurs during the consolidation phase of therapy, after autologous stem cell transplant (ASCT) and prior to maintenance with immunotherapy and retinoic acid. For patients with surgical resections of less than 90%, 5-year cumulative incidence of local progression (CILP) is up to 20%, highlighting the need for improvement.[6]

Dosages of radiotherapy have been studied over the years in an effort to improve local control, including differing radiotherapy doses based on the degree of surgical resection. Different radiotherapy methods, such as proton therapy, have also been studied with similar outcomes and potentially less damage to surrounding structures.[7,8] Standard treatment is 21.6 Gy to the preoperative tumor bed and end-induction residual MIBG-avid lesions.[9,10] A recent Phase III prospective clinical trial conducted by the COG for patients with newly diagnosed high-risk neuroblastoma hypothesized that patients who underwent incomplete surgical resection would have improved 5-year CILP with the addition of a 14.4 Gy boost in addition to the standard 21.6 Gy.

However, results showed that 5-year CILP was not significantly improved by boost radiotherapy of 14.4 Gy.[10]

Considerations for different patient groups

Paraspinal neuroblastomas, which arise from the paraspinal sympathetic ganglia, can grow into the neural foramina, resulting in spinal cord compression. Patients may present with:
- localized pain at the primary tumor site
- neuropathic pain
- localized weakness or changes in sensation.

This is considered a medical emergency. Many centers will initially attempt tumor control with chemotherapy because of long-term morbidities such as scoliosis, motor neuropathy and sensory neuropathy associated with laminectomy; however, if a tumor progresses with chemotherapy, laminectomy may be pursued for surgical decompression. Rarely, patients may be referred for external-beam radiotherapy for symptomatic relief. There are few studies to date that have compared outcomes of patients with paraspinal neuroblastoma treated with upfront laminectomy or radiotherapy compared with those treated with chemotherapy prior to surgical decompression.[11–13] However, a study from the French Society of Pediatric Oncology (NBL90) has reported that treatment with chemotherapy to reduce the size of intraspinal masses achieved improvement of partial neurological deficits and avoidance of neurosurgical decompression in many patients.[14]

Perinatal neuroblastoma. Advanced prenatal imaging enables prenatal detection of adrenal masses in neonates. Most tumors diagnosed in the perinatal period do not require surgery. ANBL00P2 is a prospective study led by the COG that included 87 infants, aged under 6 months, with small adrenal masses (< 3.2 cm for solid masses and < 5 cm for cystic masses). Of the 87 infants, 83 were initially observed. Two-thirds of patients had spontaneous reduction in tumor volume, with 27 patients having no residual mass by the end of follow-up; 81% of patients on this study were able to avoid surgery. Three-year OS was 100%. Standard of care for these patients is to observe patients with L1 tumors less than 5 cm as the vast majority will spontaneously regress. Patients with L1 tumors greater than 5 cm or L2 tumors should undergo medical treatment and/or resection, with further care based on risk stratification as described above.[15,16]

Stage MS disease. Infants with INRG stage MS disease without hepatomegaly or *MYCN* amplification, but with favorable biological markers, may also be observed by watchful waiting. Up to 70% of these patients undergo spontaneous regression of their disease.[17] Infants are stratified by INRG risk groups and are treated accordingly.

Patients with low-risk disease generally have INRGSS L1 disease without *MYCN* amplification and favorable histological features, with or without GTR of the primary tumor. Outcomes for these patients are excellent after treatment with surgical resection without any need for adjuvant chemotherapy (Figure 5.1).[18,19] In a subgroup of young patients (age <12 months) with L1 disease (maximum tumor diameter <5 cm), disease may be managed by observation alone. Low-risk disease management with observation, with or without surgical

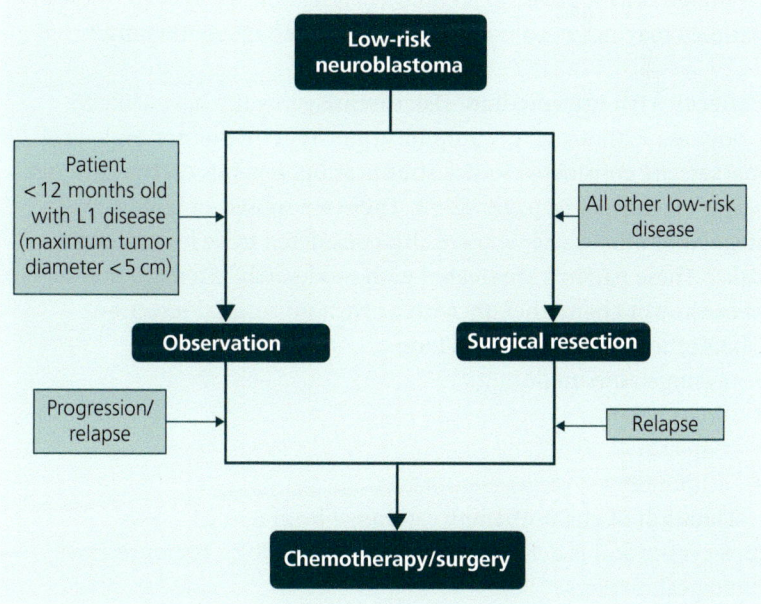

Figure 5.1 Treatment pathway for patients with low-risk neuroblastoma.

resection, was shown to be safe and effective in a non-randomized COG clinical trial (P9641) of 951 infants and children with INSS stage 2A and 2B disease. These patients, either observed after resection or given adjuvant chemotherapy (for symptomatic disease with <50% surgical removal of tumor burden or unresectable progressive disease after surgery), were found to have similar 5-year EFS (89% versus 91%) and OS (97% versus 98%).[1]

Recent reports have presented data showing that patients with low-risk disease managed by watchful observation have 5-year EFS of more than 93%. Patients who do experience relapse are subsequently treated with chemotherapy and/or additional surgery, and 5-year OS is reported to be 95%.[1,18] Watchful observation involves serial ultrasounds of the primary tumor mass along with analysis of urine catecholamines (homovanillic acid and vanillylmandelic acid). These evaluations should be performed every 3, 6, 12 and then 24 weeks for two visits each. If there is concern for an increase in tumor size, the frequency of evaluations may be increased to every 3 weeks. If tumor progression is found, surgical biopsy and resection should be undertaken if possible. If complete resection is achieved, these patients may not need further treatment with chemotherapy.[20]

Patients with intermediate-risk disease generally have INRGSS L2 disease without *MYCN* amplification. Whether or not biological markers are considered in risk stratification depends on the patient's age at diagnosis (see pages 43–8). There are subsets of patients with stage M or MS disease who are also considered to be intermediate risk.[21] These patients are treated with moderately intensive multiagent neoadjuvant chemotherapy with or without surgical resection. Chemotherapeutic agents include:
- cyclophosphamide
- doxorubicin
- cisplatin
- etoposide.

Duration of chemotherapy can range from 6 to 24 weeks (2–8 cycles) and is determined by tumor histology, response and biological markers.

A multimodal approach was found to be effective in a report from the Children's Cancer Group (CCG) in which the 4-year EFS for patients with favorable biology was 100% after treatment with 5 cycles of neoadjuvant chemotherapy followed by surgical resection, and additional cycles of chemotherapy and radiotherapy for gross residual disease. The 4-year EFS for patients with at least one unfavorable biological marker was 90%.[22] Given these results, subsequent clinical trials have focused on decreasing treatment intensity while maintaining survival rates.

SIOPEN demonstrated success in a study administering low doses of cyclophosphamide and vincristine to 180 infants with unresectable disease. Patients were given lowered doses of chemotherapy until the tumor became resectable, with 5-year EFS and OS remaining at 90% and 99%, respectively.[23]

COG study A3961 demonstrated comparable 3-year EFS and OS (88% and 96%, respectively) in patients with favorable tumor biology treated with 4 cycles of chemotherapy, while those with unfavorable tumor biology were treated with 8 cycles.[23] COG trial ANBL0531 subsequently demonstrated that patients treated with 2 cycles of chemotherapy had 3-year EFS and OS of 87% and 99%, respectively, compared with patients treated with 4 or 8 cycles (3-year EFS of 87% and 80%, and 3-year OS of 94% and 87%, respectively). Therefore, the duration of chemotherapy required is dependent on tumor biology, with more cycles warranted in patients with unfavorable histology, diploidy or SCAs.[24]

Cooperative groups now recommend the avoidance of radiotherapy for patients with intermediate-risk disease. Exceptions are in settings of life-threatening complications, organ-threatening disease, or disease progression after surgical and chemotherapeutic interventions.

Patients with high-risk disease. Generally defined by *MYCN* amplification, age greater than 18 months at diagnosis and metastatic disease (see pages 43–8), high-risk patients are at greater risk of relapsed or refractory disease and therefore require aggressive multimodal therapy. Before multimodal therapy was implemented, survival rates were as low as 15%,[25] and patients treated with high-dose therapy as per CCG protocol 3891 and COG protocol A3973 had 5-year EFS of 30–40%.[26] Subsequently, COG trial ANBL0032 demonstrated improved EFS and OS with the inclusion of immunotherapy.[27] More recently, COG trial ANBL0532 has shown the best 3-year EFS to date (63%) with intense consolidation therapy.

Standard-of-care treatment for high-risk neuroblastoma

The standard-of-care treatment regimen for high-risk neuroblastoma in the USA and Canada comprises 5 cycles of induction chemotherapy during which surgical resection is performed, consolidative myeloablative chemotherapy with ASCT followed by radiotherapy and, finally, postconsolidation immunotherapy (Figure 5.2). Survival rates for high-risk disease have improved but remain low at 50–60%.[28]

Induction

Treatment. In the USA, induction comprises neoadjuvant chemotherapy and surgical resection of the primary tumor, and its purpose is to reduce metastatic sites of disease in addition to local control of the primary tumor. Chemotherapeutic agents used during induction include:
- vincristine
- cyclophosphamide
- topotecan
- doxorubicin
- cisplatin
- etoposide.

Typically, there are 4 cycles of neoadjuvant chemotherapy, followed by surgical resection. Upon recovery from surgery, patients receive a fifth cycle of chemotherapy. Induction chemotherapy in Europe typically consists of rapid COJEC (a combination of cisplatin, vincristine, carboplatin, etoposide and cyclophosphamide given every 10 days).[29,30]

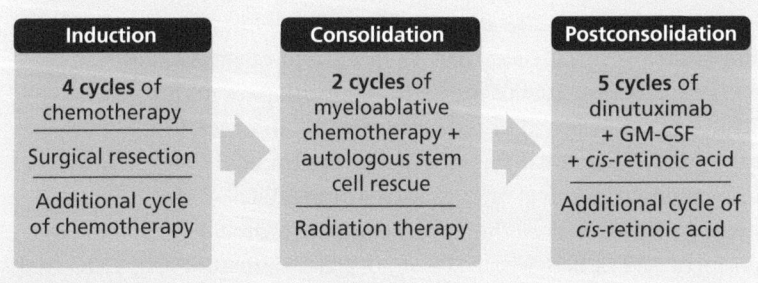

Figure 5.2 Current standard-of-care regimen for high-risk neuroblastoma. GM-CSF, granulocyte-macrophage colony-stimulating factor.

Adverse effects during induction chemotherapy include nausea, vomiting, marrow suppression, electrolyte derangements and acute kidney injury, for which supportive care is provided as needed. Long-term effects include secondary malignancy, cardiomyopathy and hearing loss (see Chapter 8).

Approaches in development. COG trial ANBL1531 (NCT03126916) is looking at the efficacy and safety of incorporating crizotinib, an ALK inhibitor, for patients with tumors positive for *ALK*-activating mutations (which represent approximately 10–15% of newly diagnosed cases of high-risk neuroblastoma).[31] Crizotinib is administered after the first cycle of induction chemotherapy until consolidation, and is then restarted after marrow recovery from myeloablative chemotherapy and ASCT. The trial was recently amended to incorporate lorlatinib instead of crizotinib.

ANBL1531 is also evaluating the use of upfront ^{131}I-MIBG therapy between the third and fourth cycles of induction chemotherapy to decrease metastatic tumor burden. ^{131}I-MIBG emits higher-energy beta and gamma radiation than ^{123}I-MIBG, which is used for imaging. Historically, ^{131}I-MIBG has been used for relapsed disease and has been shown to be effective in the treatment of cortical bone and bone marrow disease.[32]

Adding immunotherapy that targets disialoganglioside (GD2) (which is overexpressed on neuroblastoma cells) to induction chemotherapy is also being evaluated. Results from a single-center Phase II study have shown that administration of the GD2-targeted humanized monoclonal antibody hu14.18K322A during 6 cycles of induction chemotherapy significantly improved response rates and outcomes in children with newly diagnosed high-risk neuroblastoma.[33] A Phase II study (NCT05489887) is also under way to evaluate the efficacy and safety of adding the humanized GD2-directed monoclonal antibody naxitamab (see page 66) to induction chemotherapy. Meanwhile, a Phase III COG trial (NCT06172296) plans to assess the addition of the chimeric antibody dinutuximab (see page 63) in this setting.

Consolidation

Treatment begins once a patient has been shown to have stable disease, a partial response or better, as assessed by disease evaluation with ^{123}I-MIBG, CT or MRI, and bone marrow biopsy, and aims to eliminate remaining residual disease. Some institutions utilize a Curie score cut-off for proceeding with consolidation, although such practice has not been validated by prospective clinical trials and is based on retrospective studies. An end-of-induction Curie score ≤2 has been the standard cut-off for moving forward with transplant versus not, but mostly in the context of patients who received single high-dose chemotherapy and ASCT. Recent data suggest that a Curie score cut-off of 0 may be optimal for patients undergoing tandem high-dose chemotherapy and ASCT. However, this will require validation in future trials.[34]

In the USA and Canada, standard consolidation consists of 2 cycles of myeloablative chemotherapy followed by ASCT after each cycle. Patients will generally undergo peripheral stem cell collection during induction after the second cycle of chemotherapy. A prospective randomized trial undertaken by the COG demonstrated that technology used to purge the stem cell product of tumor cells was safe and did not affect outcomes.[35]

COG study ANBL0532 randomized 355 patients with high-risk neuroblastoma to either single transplant with carboplatin, etoposide and melphalan (CEM), or tandem transplants with thiotepa and cyclophosphamide followed by reduced-dose CEM. The results demonstrated improved 3-year EFS (63% versus 49%) but similar 3-year OS in the cohort that received tandem transplants compared with those who received a single transplant. However, for the subset of patients who received immunotherapy after tandem transplant, both EFS and OS were significantly improved (EFS 73.3% vs 54.7%, OS 84% vs 73.5%).[36] Therefore, standard-of-care treatment and the most recent COG protocol (ANBL1531) incorporate tandem transplants in consolidation therapy.

Alternatively, there are cooperative groups that continue to perform single ASCT after 1 cycle of myeloablative chemotherapy. In HR-NBL1, a SIOPEN Phase III trial, 600 patients with high-risk neuroblastoma were given myeloablative chemotherapy with either busulfan and melphalan, or CEM preceding ASCT. Patients who received busulfan and melphalan had significantly improved 3-year EFS (50% versus 38%) and 5-year OS (54% vs 41%).[37] Most institutions perform ASCT. Although single-institution outcomes after omitting high-dose chemotherapy/ASCT between induction chemotherapy and postconsolidation anti-GD2 antibody therapy have been similar, results have not been examined in a prospective clinical trial across multiple institutions.[38]

Once marrow recovery is complete after ASCT, patients receive radiotherapy to the primary tumor site (see pages 55–6) as well as any metastatic sites identified by MIBG imaging at the end of induction therapy. Radiation boost to gross residual disease is no longer recommended after COG study ANBL0532 showed no improvement in 5-year CILP.[10,38]

Adverse effects observed include severe mucositis, liver toxicities (hepatitis and sinusoidal obstruction syndrome), infection and acute kidney injury. These complications are often successfully treated with supportive care. However, it is important to continue monitoring patients for late effects (see pages 96–7).

Postconsolidation

Treatment. Postconsolidation or maintenance is the final phase of therapy. It is focused on eliminating residual disease with immunotherapy targeted against GD2. Patients with high-risk disease in the USA receive 5 cycles of dinutuximab, a US Food and Drug Administration (FDA)-approved chimeric antibody that targets GD2, which is given with the cytokine GM-CSF (granulocyte-macrophage colony-stimulating factor) in addition to *cis*-retinoic acid. This is followed by a course of *cis*-retinoic acid alone, which works by promoting neuroblastoma cell differentiation.[27,39]

Dinutuximab-beta is a chimeric monoclonal antibody (mAb) against GD2 with a longer and slower infusion rate than dinutuximab. It retains regulatory approval in Europe, but not in the USA. It was used in a SIOPEN trial that studied its use with the addition of interleukin-2 (IL-2); however, increased toxicity was seen without improved outcomes, resulting in the removal of IL-2 from existing studies with dinutuximab and dinutuximab-beta.[40]

Adverse effects. Because GD2 is also expressed on peripheral nerves, one of the major side effects of dinutuximab is neuropathic pain. Therefore, patients are started on continuous morphine before initiation of dinutuximab infusion. Other adverse effects include capillary leak syndrome due to increased inflammation; therefore, it is important to monitor patients' fluid status, urine output and serum albumin levels. Supportive care with albumin boluses and/or furosemide is provided as needed while patients receive dinutuximab.

Post-therapy relapse prevention

Recently, the FDA approved eflornithine (DFMO), an ornithine decarboxylase inhibitor, to reduce the risk of relapse in adult and pediatric patients with high-risk neuroblastoma who have demonstrated at least a partial response to prior multiagent, multimodal therapy, including anti-GD2 immunotherapy.

In a single-arm Phase II study (NCT02395666), patients received up to 2 years of eflornithine therapy. Outcomes were compared with historical survival rates for patients treated in the immunotherapy arm of COG study ANBL0032 (see page 59). Four-year EFS for patients treated with eflornithine was 84% versus 72% for the historical controls. Patients treated with eflornithine also had improved 4-year OS compared with those who did not receive eflornithine (96% vs 84%).[41]

Refractory and relapsed neuroblastoma

Patients who have refractory or relapsed disease remain challenging to treat and have a poor prognosis. Of the approximately 50% of patients who relapse or fail to respond to initial therapy, the long-term survival rate is 20%.[42] Recurrence most often occurs at the primary site of disease, cortical bone, bone marrow and the liver. It is rare in the CNS or lungs, and patients are often referred for clinical trials because of limited standard treatment options.

Dinutuximab, irinotecan and temozolomide. COG trial ANBL1221 (NCT01767194) studied the efficacy of adding dinutuximab versus temsirolimus to the chemotherapeutic agents irinotecan and temozolomide for the treatment of patients with neuroblastoma at first relapse or progression, and refractory disease. Clinical response was seen for 42% of patients treated with dinutuximab, irinotecan and temozolomide, while patients treated with temsirolimus, irinotecan and temozolomide had a response rate of 6%.[43] Therefore, salvage therapy with dinutuximab, irinotecan and temozolomide is considered for many patients whose disease is refractory, relapsed or progressive.

Iodine-131-meta-iodobenzylguanidine has been used to treat patients with relapsed or refractory neuroblastoma for nearly 40 years.[44] As an analog of norepinephrine, MIBG is selectively taken up by sympathetic nervous tissue and nearly 90% of neuroblastomas. When formulated with ^{131}I, it becomes a radionucleotide for the treatment of neuroblastoma.

Treatment. Objective response rates up to 40% have been seen with doses greater than 12 mCi/kg, with the typical dose used being 15–18 mCi/kg.[45] ^{131}I-MIBG has been studied both alone and in combination with chemotherapy for patients with relapsed or refractory neuroblastoma.[44-47] A recent Phase II trial conducted by the New Approaches to Neuroblastoma Therapy (NANT) consortium showed that patients who received a combination of ^{131}I-MIBG and vorinostat had significantly higher response rates after one treatment course than patients who received either ^{131}I-MIBG alone or in combination with vincristine and irinotecan.[46] Given the activity of ^{131}I-MIBG in the relapsed and refractory setting, it has also been evaluated in the upfront treatment of high-risk neuroblastoma and has been shown to be safe when given during the induction phase of treatment.[48] Whether or not the addition of ^{131}I-MIBG to current high-risk neuroblastoma therapy improves overall outcomes is unknown, and is a point of investigation in a currently enrolling COG trial for newly diagnosed patients (NCT03126916).

Adverse effects and considerations. Myelosuppression, most notably thrombocytopenia, is the main toxicity experienced following treatment with ^{131}I-MIBG. Up to 50% of patients who receive doses at or equal to 15 mCi/kg need an ASCT.[49] It is standard practice to ensure that adequate stem cell support is available for infusion, usually for 14 days after ^{131}I-MIBG therapy. Growth factor support is also administered as needed. Non-hematologic toxicities are rare. Given the high level of radioactivity of ^{131}I-MIBG, US patients must remain in radiation isolation following infusion until their radiation emissions meet State clearance regulations, typically around 5 days. Patients also receive potassium iodide as thyroid protection and a Foley catheter for bladder protection.[49] Younger patients often need to receive sedation while they are at their highest level of radiation, because it is exceedingly difficult for a young child to be separated from their caregiver while in radiation isolation.[50] Administration of ^{131}I-MIBG requires specialist hospital infrastructure to safely administer this potent radionucleotide. Because of this, only a handful of ^{131}I-MIBG centers exist in the USA, potentially complicating access to this specialized treatment.

Naxitamab-gqgk is a humanized mAb against GD2 (also known as hu3F8). Based on preliminary results of Phase II studies (NCT03363373 and NCT01757626), it was granted accelerated approval by the FDA for the treatment of patients aged 1 year or older with relapsed or refractory high-risk neuroblastoma in the bone or bone marrow who have demonstrated a partial response, minor response or stable disease before therapy initiation with naxitamab-gqgk.[51] In a pre-planned interim analysis, 50% of patients responded to naxitamab.[52]

Because patients with relapsed or refractory high-risk neuroblastoma may also have soft tissue metastases, naxitamab-gqgk with GMCSF is also being investigated in combination with irinotecan and temozolomide in patients with primary refractory or relapsed disease (NCT04560166); response rates of 37–47% have been reported with this regimen.[53,54] Naxitamab is also being investigated with isotretinoin in patients with high-risk neuroblastoma in first remission (NCT04909515) and in combination with induction therapy for patients with newly diagnosed high-risk neuroblastoma (NCT05489887).

Adoptive immunotherapy uses chimeric antigen receptor (CAR) T-cell therapy. CAR T cells are engineered from the patient's own T cells to express an extracellular domain that targets a specific tumor antigen. Binding of the CAR T cell to its target antigen results in activation of its intracellular domain, which is adapted from the T-cell receptor CD3z domain. This results in CAR T-cell cytotoxicity against cells expressing the target antigen. CAR T-cell therapy has been successful in the treatment of relapsed and refractory B-cell malignancies. Research to identify ideal tumor antigens that are expressed specifically on solid tumors such as neuroblastoma is ongoing. Early-phase clinical trials studying the efficacy and safety of CAR T-cell products against two different tumor antigens expressed on neuroblastoma cells, GD2 (NCT03635632)[55] and CD276 (also known as B7H3; NCT04483778),[56] are under way.

Recovery and post-treatment care

Patients with intermediate-risk neuroblastoma will often have a central venous catheter placed by the surgical team for use during treatment with chemotherapy. Once local control and remission is confirmed by imaging and laboratory analyses, these are promptly removed to decrease the risk of catheter-associated thrombus and infection. Patients typically remain on *Pneumocystis jiroveci* pneumonia prophylaxis for 3 to 6 months (depending on the duration of chemotherapy) after the completion of therapy. Any live vaccines that could not be given during therapy may be given from 6 months after therapy. Long-term surveillance is continued:
- every 3 months for 6 months
- then every 6 months until 24 months off therapy
- then every 12 months until 36 months off therapy.[57]

Patients with high-risk neuroblastoma will similarly undergo central venous catheter removal once remission is confirmed. *P. jiroveci* pneumonia prophylaxis is typically continued for 6 months after therapy. Resumption of live vaccines is deferred until the patient is at least 6 months off therapy. Laboratory evaluations including CBCs, electrolytes, renal function and hepatic function are obtained every 3 months for 1 year, followed by every 6 months the following year and then annually after that. Endocrine laboratory analyses such as thyroid function, hemoglobin A1c and female reproductive hormones (follicle-stimulating hormone, luteinizing hormone and anti-Müllerian hormone) are obtained at the end of therapy, and as needed afterwards. Echocardiograms to monitor heart function are conducted annually. Surveillance imaging is obtained:
- every 3 months for 6 months
- then every 6 months until 24 months off therapy
- then every 12 months until 36 months off therapy.[57]

Palliative care

Given the aggressive nature of high-risk neuroblastoma and the intensity of therapy, it is often beneficial to engage palliative care early on in treatment. Contrary to the common belief that palliative care is equivalent to end-of-life care, its role is flexible and focuses on improving quality of life regardless of prognosis. Palliative support can range from pain control and treatment of chemotherapy-induced nausea and vomiting, to facilitating conversations to address the emotional tolls of chronic illness. In cases of relapsed or refractory disease, the palliative care team also helps guide discussions regarding goals of care as they evolve. They become a crucial part of the medical team, often serving as a bridge of communication between the patient and the oncology team.

Key points – management

- The goals of surgery are to establish diagnosis, determine accurate staging, and conduct the most complete surgical resection that preserves organ function and avoids disability. Thoracic neuroblastomas are characterized by generally more favorable biology and better survival rates than abdominal and pelvic tumors, and surgical resection is often curative.
- Neuroblastoma arising from the paraspinal sympathetic ganglia can grow into the neural foramina, resulting in spinal cord compression. Patients present with localized pain at the primary tumor site, neuropathic pain, and localized weakness or changes in sensation. This is considered a medical emergency.
- Of infants with stage MS disease without hepatomegaly or *MYCN* amplification, with favorable biological markers, 70% undergo spontaneous regression of disease and may be treated with watchful waiting.
- Low-risk neuroblastoma may be treated by watchful waiting or surgical resection (depending on risk factors such as age at diagnosis and tumor size).
- Duration of chemotherapy for treatment of intermediate-risk neuroblastoma can range from 6 to 24 weeks (2–8 cycles). This is determined by response, tumor histology and biological markers.

CONTINUED

Key points – management *(CONTD)*

- High-risk neuroblastoma treatment comprises induction chemotherapy and surgical resection, consolidative myeloablative chemotherapy with ASCT, radiotherapy and postconsolidation immunotherapy with dinutuximab, GM-CSF and *cis*-retinoic acid.
- There are many ongoing clinical trials focused on treatment and improving survival in newly diagnosed and relapsed and refractory neuroblastoma. The need to reduce toxicity while maintaining outcomes is also a key research focus.
- It is important to involve palliative care early on during treatment for patients with high-risk neuroblastoma for additional support in pain management, as well as end-of-life discussions.

References

1. Strother DR, London WB, Schmidt ML et al. Outcome after surgery alone or with restricted use of chemotherapy for patients with low-risk neuroblastoma: results of Children's Oncology Group study P9641. *J Clin Oncol* 2012;30:1842–8.
2. Overman RE, Kartal TT, Cunningham RJ et al. Optimization of percutaneous biopsy for diagnosis and pretreatment risk assessment of neuroblastoma. *Ped Blood Cancer* 2020;67:e28153.
3. La Quaglia MP, Kushner BH, Su W et al. The impact of gross total resection on local control and survival in high-risk neuroblastoma. *J Pediatr Surg* 2004;39:412–17.
4. Malek MM, Mollen KP, Kane TD et al. Thoracic neuroblastoma: a retrospective review of our institutional experience with comparison of the thoracoscopic and open approaches to resection. *J Pediatr Surg* 2010;45:1622–26.
5. DeCou JM, Schlatter MG, Mitchell DS. Primary thoracoscopic gross total resection of neuroblastoma. *J Laparoendosc Adv Surg Tech A* 2005;15:470–3.
6. Fischer J, Pohl A, Volland R et al. Complete surgical resection improves outcome in INRG high-risk patients with localized neuroblastoma older than 18 months. *BMC Cancer* 2017;17:520.

7. Bagley AF, Grosshans DR, Philip NV et al. Efficacy of proton therapy in children with high-risk and locally recurrent neuroblastoma. *Pediatr Blood Cancer* 2019; 66:e27786.
8. Hill-Kayser CE, Tochner Z, Li Y et al. Outcomes after proton therapy for treatment of pediatric high-risk neuroblastoma. *Int J Radiat Oncol Biol Phys* 2019;104:401–8.
9. Haas-Kogan DA, Swift PS, Selch M et al. Impact of radiotherapy for high-risk neuroblastoma: a Children's Cancer Group study. *Int J Radiat Oncol Biol Phys* 2003;56:28–39.
10. Liu KX, Naranjo A, Zhang FF et al. Prospective evaluation of radiation dose escalation in patients with high-risk neuroblastoma and gross residual disease after surgery: a report from the Children's Oncology Group ANBL0532 study. *J Clin Oncol* 2020;38:2741–52.
11. Hoover M, Bowman LC, Crawford SE et al. Long-term outcome of patients with intraspinal neuroblastoma. *Med Pediatr Oncol* 1999;32: 353–9.
12. Katzenstein HM, Kent PM, London WB, Cohn SL. Treatment and outcome of 83 children with intraspinal neuroblastoma: the Pediatric Oncology Group experience. *J Clin Oncol* 2001;19:1047–55.
13. Kraal K, Blom T, Tytgat L et al. Neuroblastoma with intraspinal extension: health problems in long-term survivors. *Pediatr Blood Cancer* 2016;63:990–6.
14. Plantaz D, Rubie H, Michon J et al. The treatment of neuroblastoma with intraspinal extension with chemotherapy followed by surgical removal of residual disease. A prospective study of 42 patients – results of the NBL 90 study of the French Society of Pediatric Oncology. *Cancer* 1996;78:311–19.
15. Brodeur G, Hogarty M, Bagatell R et al. Neuroblastoma. In: Pizzo PA, Poplack DG, eds. *Principles and Practice of Pediatric Oncology*, 7th edition. Wolters Kluwer, 2016.
16. Davidoff A. Neonatal neuroblastoma. *Clin Perinatol* 2021;48:101–15.
17. Tas ML, Nagtegaal M, Kraal KCJM et al. Neuroblastoma stage 4S: tumor regression rate and risk factors of progressive disease. *Pediatr Blood Cancer* 2020;67:e28061.
18. Perez C, Matthay K, Atkinson J et al. Biologic variables in the outcome of stages I and II neuroblastoma treated with surgery as primary therapy: a Children's Cancer Group Study. *J Clin Oncol* 2000;18:18–26.
19. De Bernardi B, Mosseri V, Rubie H et al. Treatment of localised resectable neuroblastoma. Results of the LNESG1 study by the SIOP Europe Neuroblastoma Group. *Br J Cancer* 2008;99:1027–33.

20. Interiano R, Davidoff A. Current management of neonatal neuroblastoma. *Curr Pediatr Rev* 2015;11:179.
21. Nickerson HJ, Matthay K, Seeger RC et al. Favorable biology and outcome of stage IV-S neuroblastoma with supportive care or minimal therapy: a Children's Cancer Group study. *J Clin Oncol* 2000;18:477–86.
22. Matthay KK, Perez C, Seeger RC et al. Successful treatment of stage III neuroblastoma based on prospective biologic staging: a Children's Cancer Group study. *J Clin Oncol* 1998;16:1256–64.
23. Baker DL, Schmidt ML, Cohn SL et al. Outcome after reduced chemotherapy for intermediate-risk neuroblastoma. *N Engl J Med* 2010;363:1313–23.
24. Twist CJ, Schmidt ML, Naranjo A et al. Maintaining outstanding outcomes using response- and biology-based therapy for intermediate-risk neuroblastoma: a report from the Children's Oncology Group study ANBL0531. *J Clin Oncol* 2019;37:3243–55.
25. Matthay KK, Villablanca JG, Seeger RC et al. Treatment of high-risk neuroblastoma with intensive chemotherapy, radiotherapy, autologous bone marrow transplantation, and 13-*cis*-retinoic acid. *N Engl J Med* 1999;341:1165–73.
26. von Allmen D, Davidoff AM, London WB et al. Impact of extent of resection on local control and survival in patients from the COG A3973 study with high-risk neuroblastoma. *J Clin Oncol* 2017;35:208–16.
27. Yu AL, Gilman AL, Ozkaynak MF et al. Anti-GD2 antibody with GM-CSF, interleukin-2, and isotretinoin for neuroblastoma. *N Engl J Med* 2010;363:1324–34.
28. Coughlan D, Gianferante M, Lynch CF et al. Treatment and survival of childhood neuroblastoma: evidence from a population-based study in the United States. *Pediatr Hematol Oncol* 2017;34:320–30.
29. Ladenstein R, Valteau-Couanet D, Brock P et al. Randomized trial of prophylactic granulocyte colony-stimulating factor during rapid COJEC induction in pediatric patients with high-risk neuroblastoma: the European HR-NBL1/SIOPEN study. *J Clin Oncol* 2010;28:3516–24.
30. Pearson AD, Pinkerton CR, Lewis IJ et al. High-dose rapid and standard induction chemotherapy for patients aged over 1 year with stage 4 neuroblastoma: a randomised trial. *Lancet Oncol* 2008;9:247–56.
31. Bellini A, Pötschger U, Bernard V et al. Frequency and prognostic impact of *ALK* amplifications and mutations in the European Neuroblastoma Study Group (SIOPEN) High-Risk Neuroblastoma Trial (HR-NBL1). *J Clin Oncol* 2021;39:3377–90.

32. Kayano D, Kinuya S. Current consensus on I-131 MIBG therapy. *Nucl Med Mol Imaging* 2018;52:254–65.
33. Furman WL, McCarville B, Shulkin BL, et al. Improved outcomes in children with newly diagnosed high risk neuroblastoma treated with chemoimmunotherapy: updated results of a Phase II study using hu14.18K322A. *J Clin Oncol* 2022;40:335–344.
34. Streby KA, Parisi MT, Shulkin BL, et al. Impact of diagnostic and end-of-induction Curie scores with tandem high-dose chemotherapy and autologous transplants for metastatic high-risk neuroblastoma: A report from the Children's Oncology Group. *Pediatr Blood Cancer* 2023;70:e30418.
35. Kreissman SG, Seeger RC, Matthay KK et al. Purged versus non-purged peripheral blood stem-cell transplantation for high-risk neuroblastoma (COG A3973): a randomised phase 3 trial. *Lancet Oncol* 2013;14: 999–1008.
36. Park JR, Kreissman SG, London WB et al. Effect of tandem autologous stem cell transplant vs single transplant on event-free survival in patients with high-risk neuroblastoma. *JAMA* 2019;322:746–55.
37. Ladenstein R, Pötschger U, Pearson ADJ et al. Busulfan and melphalan versus carboplatin, etoposide, and melphalan as high-dose chemotherapy for high-risk neuroblastoma (HR-NBL1/SIOPEN): an international, randomised, multi-arm, open-label, phase 3 trial. *Lancet Oncol* 2017;18:500–14.
38. Kushner BH, Ostrovnaya I, Cheung IY et al. Lack of survival advantage with autologous stem-cell transplantation in high-risk neuroblastoma consolidated by anti-GD2 immunotherapy and isotretinoin. *Oncotarget* 2016;7:4155–66.
39. Matthay KK, Reynolds CP, Seeger RC et al. Long-term results for children with high-risk neuroblastoma treated on a randomized trial of myeloablative therapy followed by 13-*cis*-retinoic acid: a Children's Oncology Group study. *J Clin Oncol* 2009;27:1007–13.
40. Ladenstein R, Pötschger U, Valteau-Couanet D et al. Interleukin 2 with anti-GD2 antibody ch14.18/CHO (dinutuximab beta) in patients with high-risk neuroblastoma (HR-NBL1/SIOPEN): a multicentre, randomised, phase 3 trial. *Lancet Oncol* 2018;19:1617–29.

41. Oesterheld J, Ferguson W, Kraveka JM, et al. Eflornithine as postimmunotherapy maintenance in high-risk neuroblastoma: externally controlled, propensity score-matched survival outcome comparisons. *J Clin Oncol* 2024;42:90–102.
42. DuBois SG, Macy ME, Henderson TO. High-risk and relapsed neuroblastoma: toward more cures and better outcomes. *Am Soc Clin Oncol Educ Book* 2022;42:1–13.
43. Mody R, Naranjo A, Van Ryn C et al. Irinotecan–temozolomide with temsirolimus or dinutuximab in children with refractory or relapsed neuroblastoma (COG ANBL1221): an open-label, randomised, phase 2 trial. *Lancet Oncol* 2017;18:946–57.
44. DuBois SG, Matthay KK. Radiolabeled metaiodobenzylguanidine for the treatment of neuroblastoma. *Nucl Med Biol* 2008;35(suppl 1):S35–48.
45. Matthay KK, Yanik G, Messina J et al. Phase II study on the effect of disease sites, age, and prior therapy on response to iodine-131-metaiodobenzylguanidine therapy in refractory neuroblastoma. *J Clin Oncol* 2007;25:1054–60.
46. DuBois SG, Granger MM, Groshen S et al. Randomized phase II trial of MIBG versus MIBG, vincristine, and irinotecan versus MIBG and vorinostat for patients with relapsed or refractory neuroblastoma: a report from NANT Consortium. *J Clin Oncol* 2021;39:3506–14.
47. McCluskey AG, Boyd M, Pimlott SL et al. Experimental treatment of neuroblastoma using [^{131}I]meta-iodobenzyl-guanidine and topotecan in combination. *Br J Radiol* 2008;81:S28–35.
48. Weiss BD, Yanik G, Naranjo A et al. A safety and feasibility trial of ^{131}I-MIBG in newly diagnosed high-risk neuroblastoma: a Children's Oncology Group study. *Pediatr Blood Cancer* 2021;68:e29117.
49. DuBois SG, Messina J, Maris JM et al. Hematologic toxicity of high-dose iodine-131-metaiodobenzylguanidine therapy for advanced neuroblastoma. *J Clin Oncol* 2004;22:2452–60.
50. Lee JS, Wu R, Wong T et al. Extended sedation with continuous midazolam or dexmedetomidine infusion for young children receiving ^{131}I-MIBG radiopharmaceutical therapy for advanced neuroblastoma. *Pediatr Blood Cancer* 2016;63:471–8.
51. Markham A. Naxitamab: first approval. *Drugs* 2021;81:291–6.

52. Mora J, Chan GC, Morgenstern DA et al. Patterns of improvement following initial response in patients treated with naxitamab for relapsed/refractory high-risk neuroblastoma. *J Clin Oncol* 2024;42(16_suppl):10033.
53. Modak S, Kushner BH, Mauguen A et al. Naxitamab-based chemoimmunotherapy for resistant high-risk neuroblastoma: results of "HITS" phase II study. *J Clin Oncol.* 2022;40(16_suppl):10028.
54. Mora J, Castaneda A, Gorostegui M et al. Naxitamab combined with granulocyte-macrophage colony-stimulating factor as consolidation for high-risk neuroblastoma patients in first complete remission under compassionate use–updated outcome report. *Cancers.* 2023;15:2535.
55. Omer B. *Phase I Study of Autologous T Lymphocytes Expressing GD2-Specific Chimeric Antigen and Constitutively Active IL-7 Receptors for the Treatment of Patients With Relapsed or Refractory Neuroblastoma and Other GD2 Positive Solid Cancers (GAIL-N)*, 2021. clinicaltrials.gov/ct2/show/NCT03635632, last accessed 11 May 2022.
56. Park J. *Phase I Study of B7H3 CAR T Cell Immunotherapy for Recurrent/Refractory Solid Tumors in Children and Young Adults,* 2021. clinicaltrials.gov/ct2/show/NCT04483778, last accessed 11 May 2022.
57. Friedman DN, Henderson TO. Late effects and survivorship issues in patients with neuroblastoma. *Children* 2018;5:107.

6 Health disparities

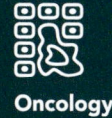
Oncology

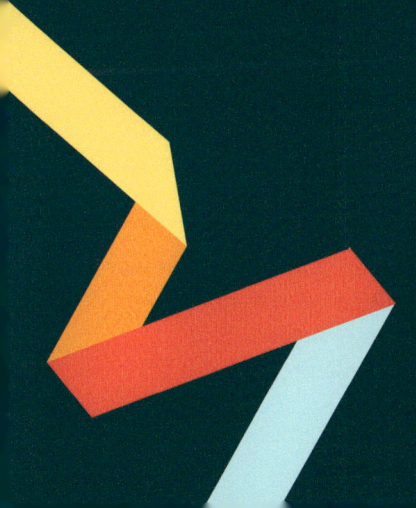

HEALTHCARE

Modern treatment strategies, tailored according to risk, have led to improved outcomes in patients with neuroblastoma. However, there are disparities in diagnosis, treatment and outcome with respect to ethnicity and socioeconomic status (SES).

Race and ethnicity

As noted in Chapter 1, Black and Native American patients in the USA have a relatively high prevalence of high-risk neuroblastoma. Disparities in diagnosis, risk status and outcome are most pronounced between Black and White children. The following findings were recorded among over 3500 patients enrolled in the COG neuroblastoma biology study in the USA.[1]

- Compared with White children, Black children were diagnosed at an older age and had greater prevalence of stage 4 disease and tumors with unfavorable histology (all $p<0.001$).
- Black (but not Hispanic or Asian) children were more likely to present with high-risk disease than White children (57% versus 44%; $p<0.001$), although there was no difference in the frequency of *MYCN* amplification or diploidy between groups.
- Black children had significantly poorer EFS than White children, as did Native American children ($p≤0.01$).
- Among high-risk patients who remained event free for at least 2 years, there was greater prevalence of late-occurring events among Black children than among White children (hazard ratio [HR] = 1.5; 95% confidence interval [CI] 1.0, 2.3; $p=0.04$).
- In accordance with the greater prevalence of high-risk disease and EFS, Black children also had significantly worse OS than White children ($p<0.001$).[1]

An analysis from the population-based SEER cancer registry, which included 1901 patients with neuroblastoma, similarly found that White children (aged 0–19 years) had a significant survival advantage over Black and Hispanic children.[2] However, the most recent analysis of the SEER registry, using data from a broader group of patients diagnosed between 1973 and 2015 (n = 2119), showed no significant association between race and survival for patients with neuroblastoma. Because this analysis included more recent patient cases than previous studies, particularly from 2010 onwards, the study suggests that improvements in treatment may have led to a lessening of racial disparities in neuroblastoma survival in recent years, and also suggests that social determinants may underlie disparities.[3] There is a call for further studies in this area to enable the provision of equitable care to all patients.

Socioeconomic status

Studies have shown that cancer survival may be influenced by SES. Factors that are closely linked to SES include early diagnosis, ease of accessing healthcare and being able to maintain treatment adherence.[4]

Although a COG study in patients with neuroblastoma recently found that every patient assessed had at least some form of health insurance, and that there was no significant difference in mortality based on the type of insurance held,[3] it remains that many patients and parents have only modest insurance coverage coupled with an income level that limits their ability to pay out-of-pocket healthcare costs.[5]

In the USA, SES of children with cancer is closely linked to race and ethnicity: for example, studies have shown that among children with acute lymphoblastic leukemia, Black patients are relatively less likely to have private insurance (34% versus 57%) and more likely to have public insurance (54% versus 23%) than White patients, parents of Hispanic and Black children are more likely to have received lower levels of high school education and live in homes with lower household incomes (each $p<0.001$) than those of White children, and lower SES is associated with worse outcome.[4] An analysis of SEER data showed that the influence of SES, though variable between cancers, can account for a large proportion of the differences in survival reported between racial groups, including almost 50% of the difference between Black or Hispanic versus White children for neuroblastoma.[2]

Socioeconomic factors that affect outcomes. Studies are under way to assess the impact of evidence-based, poverty-targeted interventions in pediatric oncology, recognizing that poverty is associated with inferior psychosocial outcomes, higher rates of relapse and decreased OS in children with cancer (NCT03638453).[6]

Poverty in children with high-risk neuroblastoma (n=371) treated in targeted immunotherapy trials in the USA was linked to poor EFS and OS in a COG analysis. In multivariable Cox regressions (adjusted for disease and treatment factors), children with high-risk neuroblastoma exposed to household poverty experienced significantly worse EFS (HR=1.90; 95% CI 1.28, 2.82; $p=0.001$) and OS (HR=2.79; 95% CI 1.63, 4.79; $p<0.001$) than unexposed children. Neighborhood poverty was not independently associated with EFS or OS, but in post-hoc analyses, children with dual-poverty exposure (neighborhood and household poverty) had significantly worse EFS (HR=2.21; 95% CI 1.48, 3.30; $p<0.001$) and OS (HR=3.70; 95% CI 2.08, 6.59; $p<0.001$) compared with those in the unexposed group.[7]

A reduced level of parent education is one of several factors found to be associated with late diagnosis across a range of pediatric tumors, leading in turn to poorer outcomes.[8]

Lack of transportation has been identified as one of the major barriers to patients and their families receiving good-quality cancer care for the following reasons.
- The inability to meet the cost of transportation can lead to the cancellation of medical appointments.[5]
- Inability to get to the pharmacy, grocery store, health education classes, peer support meetings and other resources can hinder healthcare among patients with cancer or their families.[5]
- For parents with low SES and a child with neuroblastoma, living some distance from a tertiary pediatric cancer center may limit their access to care.

Reduced social support has also been identified as a major barrier to patients and their families receiving good-quality cancer care. Patients report that social support is not well addressed as part of their oncology care, and that many healthcare providers do not consider psychosocial support to be an integral component of quality cancer care.[6] Reduced social support in US adults is associated with patient-reported delays in seeking medical care, which in turn lead to poor health outcomes.[9]

Key points – health disparities

- Disparities in diagnosis, risk status and outcome are most pronounced between Black and White children. There is a call for further studies in this area to enable the provision of equitable care to all patients.
- Studies have shown that low SES is independently associated with poor survival in patients with neuroblastoma.
- Poverty, lack of transportation and poor social support have been identified as barriers to timely and effective healthcare in families requiring pediatric oncology care.

References

1. Henderson TO, Bhatia S, Pinto N et al. Racial and ethnic disparities in risk and survival in children with neuroblastoma: a Children's Oncology Group study. *J Clin Oncol* 2011;29:76–82.
2. Kehm RD, Spector LG, Poynter JN et al. Does socioeconomic status account for racial and ethnic disparities in childhood cancer survival? *Cancer* 2018;124:4090–7.
3. Farouk FS, Viqar OA, Sheikh Z et al. The association between race and survival among pediatric patients with neuroblastoma in the US between 1973 and 2015. *Int J Environ Res Public Health* 2020;17:5119.
4. Bhatia S. Disparities in cancer outcomes: lessons learned from children with cancer. *Pediatr Blood Cancer* 2011;56:994–1002.
5. Institute of Medicine (US) Committee on Psychosocial Services to Cancer Patients/Families in a Community Setting. The psychosocial needs of cancer patients. In: Adler NE, Page AEK (eds), *Cancer Care for the Whole Patient: Meeting Psychosocial Health Needs*. National Academies Press, 2008.
6. Umaretiya PJ, Revette A, Seo A et al. PediCARE: development of a poverty-targeted intervention for pediatric cancer. *Pediatr Blood Cancer* 2021;68:e29195.
7. Bona K, Li Y, Winestone LE et al. Poverty and targeted immunotherapy: survival in Children's Oncology Group clinical trials for high-risk neuroblastoma. *J Natl Cancer Inst* 2021;113:282–91.

8. Dang-Tan T, Franco EL. Diagnosis delays in childhood cancer: a review. *Cancer* 2007;110:703–13.

9. Reisinger MW, Moss M, Clark BJ. Is lack of social support associated with a delay in seeking medical care? A cross-sectional study of Minnesota and Tennessee residents using data from the Behavioral Risk Factor Surveillance System. *BMJ Open* 2018;8:e018139.

7 Future directions and unmet needs

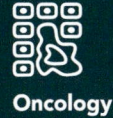
Oncology

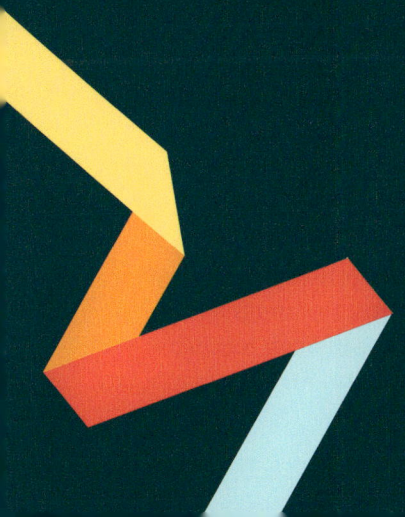

HEALTHCARE

Unmet needs in neuroblastoma

As we saw in Chapters 2–5, the prognosis and approach to treatment of neuroblastoma depend on tumor presentation, and markers such as *MYCN* amplification and genomic status. However, limitations to current treatments have been identified in several areas.

Long-term survival in high-risk patients, which comprise over 40% of patients, including children aged over 18 months with metastatic disease and those with *MYCN* amplification-positive tumors, remains low, at less than 50% at 5 years. Despite treatment, most patients experience relapse, with 5-year OS for patients with relapsed metastatic neuroblastoma of only 8%. This is despite improvements in intensive treatment, including surgery, chemotherapy, radiotherapy, high-dose therapy with ASCT, residual disease therapy and immunotherapy with mAbs against GD2.[1,2]

A lack of treatment options is problematic because the same therapeutic approach is given to all patients at presentation and treatment is only modified for patients with refractory, relapsed or progressive disease. Although molecular drivers (such as *MYCN*, *TERT*, *ATRX*, *TP53* and RAS/MAPK; see Chapter 2) have been identified for specific neuroblastoma subtypes, there are no therapies targeted directly against them as yet. This is partly due to very small patient populations that are further split into genomically defined cohorts; in addition, attention has been diverted to attempts to develop existing drugs that are already used to treat other, mostly adult, malignancies with little success.[2] Antibodies against GD2 combined with other immunomodulators (such as GM-CSF) have been an important advance (see Chapter 5), but no other new drugs have entered front-line studies for around 20 years and new options are needed.[2,3]

Treatment resistance is problematic because around 30% of patients are refractory to first-line therapy and have very poor outcomes. They are also burdened with late effects because of the intensity of their multimodal therapy.[2,3]

Improved response rate with induction chemotherapy is needed because it is ineffective in about 30% of patients. Few drugs have been introduced in this setting in recent years. Although regimens such as topotecan–vincristine–doxorubicin and irinotecan–

temozolomide–dinutuximab have yielded positive results in patients with suboptimal end-induction responses, their impacts on OS and EFS are unknown.[4] As discussed in Chapter 5, the addition of GD2-targeted therapy during induction treatment is currently being evaluated.

A lack of useful biomarkers to predict on-target effects of specific drugs has hampered drug development in neuroblastoma, and preclinical model systems that adequately reflect the nature of the disease are lacking (for example, few neuroblastoma tumor xenograft models are available).[5] The spatial and temporal heterogeneity of the disease is problematic in this regard.

Organizations and initiatives promoting cooperation in neuroblastoma research

Many consortiums and initiatives, both nationally and internationally, are dedicated to discovering and developing new treatments for patients with neuroblastoma.

Organizations

The Children's Oncology Group is a global organization with expertise in clinical development of new therapeutics for children and adolescents with cancer.

The Pediatric Early Phase Clinical Trials Network (PEP-CTN) is part of the US National Cancer Institute's program for conducting early-phase clinical trials in children with cancer. Building upon the success of the COG Phase 1 & Pilot Consortium, it is composed of 21 core COG sites in the USA and 21 non-core sites in the USA, Canada and Australia.

The New Approaches to Neuroblastoma Therapy (NANT) consortium develops and conducts neuroblastoma-specific early-phase clinical trials with the goal of generating the necessary safety and efficacy data for new agents to be incorporated into large, Phase III clinical trials.

The Beat Childhood Cancer Research Consortium offers an international network of early-phase clinical trials for patients with neuroblastoma.

The International Society of Paediatric Oncology (SIOP) is a global society, with over 2600 members worldwide, that is dedicated to designing and implementing clinical trials for pediatric and adolescent cancer.

Initiatives

The Neuroblastoma New Drug Development Strategy is an initiative started in 2012, based in Europe but now extending to North America, that is attempting to address problems in neuroblastoma research by identifying high-priority targets and coordinating clinical trials. It identified several high-priority areas for drug discovery and improvement in a published statement (Table 7.1). Another priority is to improve the strategy for conducting trials in neuroblastoma, because the wide range of clinical trials with differing treatment combinations and permutations requires a high degree of international collaboration.[6]

The Pediatric Oncology Platform was initiated in 2015 to promote initiatives developing drugs relevant to several specific pediatric oncology targets and the repositioning of existing drugs that have not been fully developed in adults. It initiated a strategy to prioritize potential pediatric indications and established a forum, ACCELERATE,

TABLE 7.1

High-priority areas identified by the Neuroblastoma New Drug Development Strategy[6]

- Strategies to develop drugs targeting TERT, telomere maintenance, ATRX, ALT, BRIP1 and RRM2, as well as direct targeting of MYC-N
- Promising preclinical data support the targeting of ALT by ATM or PARP inhibition
- Drugs targeting CDK2/9, CDK7, ATR and telomere maintenance should enter pediatric clinical development rapidly
- Optimizing the response to anti-GD2 by combinations with chemotherapy, targeted agents and other immunologic targets

ALT, alanine aminotransferase; ATM, ATM serine/threonine kinase; ATR, ataxia telangiectasia and Rad3-related protein; ATRX, ATRX chromatin remodeller; BRIP1, BRCA1-interacting helicase 1; CDK, cyclin-dependent kinase; PARP, poly(ADP-ribose) polymerase; RRM2, ribonucleotide reductase regulatory subunit M2; TERT, telomerase reverse transcriptase.

that aims to promote innovation in new drug development by bringing together clinicians, academics, patient advocates, representatives of pharmaceutical companies and regulators.[7]

Drugs and strategies in development

Many promising targets and drugs have been identified in preclinical studies, and many of these have been, or are being, explored in clinical trials focused on neuroblastoma (>500 are registered at clinicaltrials.gov). However, most agents are in Phase I development, and only a small number of agents are in Phase III trials.

Genomic studies. To ensure accurate diagnoses for individual patients and to fully personalize therapy, high-throughput genomic technologies have become prominent in neuroblastoma research. Genomic data including amplifications, deletions, point mutations and messenger RNA expression profiles (transcriptome analysis) are being used to stratify patients and guide decisions in clinical trials.[8] As the diagnosis and treatment landscape changes, these studies will provide information regarding risk stratification that will need to be built into future consensus statements and guidelines.

The Neuroblastoma Precision Medicine clinical trial established through the NANT consortium (NCT02868268) aims to develop tissue sampling and DNA-sequencing technology using a standardized gene panel that is specific for neuroblastoma (assessing *MYCN* amplification and *ALK* mutation, among other markers). It also aims to identify potential novel biomarkers.

The Next Generation Personalized Neuroblastoma Therapy study (NCT02780128) is using tumor biopsies and next-generation sequencing data to determine genetic changes that occur in patients receiving therapy. Studies such as this will help to define clonally acquired, oncogenic changes in relapsed neuroblastomas, including those that arise under the selective pressure of cytotoxic chemotherapy, potentially allowing the development of targeted therapies and new drug combinations that are directed towards aberrantly regulated pathways in relapsed disease.[9]

Targeted therapies. Many targeted agents are in development, despite the relative paucity of common somatic mutations or activated oncogenes in neuroblastoma (see pages 23–4). MYC-N has proved to be a challenging target because its DNA-binding domain lacks surfaces to which drugs might bind. However, modulation of MYC-N may be possible by targeting other pathways, such as the PI3K/protein kinase B/mammalian target of rapamycin pathway, which appears to play a role in MYC-N stabilization,[10] and downstream targets such as ornithine decarboxylase, the rate-limiting enzyme in polyamine biosynthesis. Small-molecule targeted agents include tyrosine kinase inhibitors, many of which have been used successfully in tumor types other than neuroblastoma, and agents directed against the cell cycle-controlling cyclin-dependent kinases, which are often dysregulated in cancer.

Anaplastic lymphoma kinase inhibitors. The main ALK inhibitors are listed below. In future clinical trials, it is hoped that combination strategies with conventional chemotherapy and/or other targeted therapies may overcome resistance to current ALK inhibitors.

Crizotinib, the ALK inhibitor most extensively studied in neuroblastoma, also inhibits mesenchymal epithelial transition kinase activity and is approved by the FDA for use in adult patients with *ALK*-translocated non-small cell lung cancer.[10] Phase II data from a study where crizotinib, 280 mg/m^2 once daily, was given to patients with neuroblastoma showed responses in 3 patients, with an overall response rate (ORR) of 15%. All three responding patients had ALK Arg1275Gln mutations (the most common *ALK* hotspot mutation seen in neuroblastoma and predicted to be sensitive to ALK inhibition with crizotinib). Decreased neutrophil count was the most common adverse effect.[11] Crizotinib is being evaluated in the ongoing COG ANBL1531 Phase III trial (NCT03126916).

Ceritinib, a second-generation ALK inhibitor, has shown promising results in a Phase I study. The recommended dosage in children was established as 500 mg/m^2 once daily with food. An ORR of 20% has been reported for the subset of patients with neuroblastoma.[12]

Repotrectinib (TPX-0005, a third-generation ALK inhibitor in Phase II trials), targets the active kinase conformations of ALK, c-ros oncogene 1 (ROS1) and NTRK1–3, impedes proliferation and prompts apoptosis in ALK-addicted neuroblastoma cells, and inhibits ALK-driven neurite outgrowth prompting tumor regression.[13]

Lorlatinib is a selective ATP-competitive inhibitor of ALK and ROS1 tyrosine kinases. It is in Phase III trials in patients with pediatric neuroblastoma, and is also being incorporated during induction therapy in the COG trial ANBL1531 (see page 61).

Ornithine decarboxylase inhibitors in clinical development include difluoromethylornithine, either alone (NCT02679144, NCT02395666) or in combination with etoposide (NCT01059071, NCT04301843), bortezemib (NCT02139397) or dinutuximab (NCT03794349) in high-risk patients in remission.

Targeting angiogenesis in neuroblastoma is an attractive strategy. The formation of tumor vasculature is associated with an aggressive phenotype and the overexpression of proangiogenic factors such as vascular endothelial growth factor (VEGF) correlates with high-risk disease.[14]

Bevacizumab, an antibody against VEGF, is an approved treatment for a variety of cancers. Several trials of bevacizumab in combination with other chemotherapeutic agents have been completed or are ongoing in neuroblastoma. Bevacizumab in combination with irinotecan and temozolomide for refractory and relapsed neuroblastoma (NCT01114555) did not improve response rates, and a Phase II trial of bevacizumab with cyclophosphamide and topotecan in patients with relapsed or refractory Ewing sarcoma and neuroblastoma (NCT01492673) failed to accrue enough patients for analysis. Ongoing trials in patients with relapsed or refractory neuroblastoma include bevacizumab in combination with:
- cyclophosphamide and zoledronic acid (NCT00885326)
- an anti-CD2 radioimmunoconjugate (3F8, a murine antibody against GD2 labeled with ^{123}I-MIBG) (NCT00450827)
- irinotecan, temozolomide and topotecan (BEACON; NCT02308527).[14]

Pazopanib is a multikinase inhibitor that targets VEGF receptors 1–3. It is in a clinical trial in patients with refractory neuroblastoma (NCT01130623).

Targeting epigenetic changes is of interest because the epigenetic landscape of cancer cells (for example, DNA methylation, histone modification and nucleosome remodeling) is different from that of normal cells. Histone deacetylases (HDACs) are enzymes that regulate gene expression by remodeling chromatin structure, such that aberrant histone acetylation caused by deregulated HDAC activity can promote tumor progression in neuroblastoma and other tumor types. HDAC inhibitors have been shown to inhibit tumor proliferation and induce apoptosis in preclinical neuroblastoma models.[10,15]

Vorinostat is an HDAC inhibitor that does not appear to be effective in the clinic as a single agent, but did have antitumor effects when combined with retinoids in preclinical studies of neuroblastoma. A Phase I trial in children with relapsed or refractory neuroblastoma that combined isotretinoin with vorinostat found no objective responses, but prolonged stable disease was seen in some patients with residual disease.[16] In combination with ^{123}I-MIBG, vorinostat has been shown in preclinical studies to have potential as a radiation sensitizer and promising results were recently reported from a Phase II study. Patients with relapsed or refractory neuroblastoma received one course of ^{123}I-MIBG 18 mCi/kg and ASCT 2 weeks later, plus vorinostat, 180 mg/m²/dose once daily on days 1 to 12, and showed an ORR of 32% with acceptable toxicity.[17]

Immunotherapies. Despite the low tumor mutational loads and poor immunogenic properties of neuroblastomas (such as a low rate of generation of neo-antigens), the fetal surface glycolipid GD2 has proved to be a suitable mAb-based target. Indeed, dinutuximab has become integrated into the standard of care in high-risk neuroblastoma (see page 63), in which it is thought to mediate neuroblastoma cell killing primarily through antibody-dependent cell-mediated cytotoxicity, mainly via neutrophils and natural killer (NK) cells.[18] However, the low immunogenicity of neuroblastoma has unfortunate effects because it results in a relative lack of tumor infiltration by lymphocytes, which reduces the ability of NK cells and cytotoxic T lymphocytes to kill tumor cells; therefore, different approaches from those that are applied when adults are given cancer immunotherapy may be beneficial.[18] Nevertheless, neuroblastomas express surface markers in addition to GD2 that are uncommon on mature, non-embryonic tissues, and antibodies targeting surface receptors or ligands found in the neural crest (such as ALK, CD276, CD56, L1 cell adhesion molecule [L1CAM] and polysialic acid) are being investigated.[19] Many other immunotherapy approaches are in preclinical or early clinical development in neuroblastoma, including bevacizumab (discussed earlier), the use of cancer vaccines (vaccination with tumor antigens, cytokine-producing tumor cells or dendritic cells with the aim of inducing T-cell responses), modified dendritic cells and novel combinations of immunotherapies.[18,19]

Monoclonal antibodies against GD2. Dinutuximab is a chimeric mAb that specifically targets the carbohydrate moiety of GD2. Dinutuximab has been approved by the FDA for first-line use in high-risk neuroblastoma since 2015,[20] and must be used in conjunction with 13-*cis*-retinoic acid and GM-CSF. In combination with cytotoxic compounds, dinutuximab is under further investigation in high-risk or relapsed neuroblastoma (NCT04385277 and NCT03794349).[18] Dinutuximab in combination with haploidentical NK cells is also being investigated (NCT02573896, NCT03242603, NCT02100891, NCT04211675 and NCT01807468).[18]

Naxitamab is a humanized monoclonal antibody targeting GD2 (see page 66). It has been approved by the FDA for the treatment of relapsed or refractory high-risk neuroblastoma in the bone or bone marrow (NCT03363373), and it is being studied as an addition to induction therapy for newly diagnosed high-risk neuroblastoma (NCT05489887).

Chimeric antigen receptor T cells are under investigation in numerous clinical trials for neuroblastoma, with targets including CD276 (NCT04483778), epidermal growth factor receptor (NCT03618381), GD2 (NCT02919046, NCT02765243, NCT02761915, NCT01822652, NCT03635632, NCT03721068, NCT03294954, NCT02992210, NCT03373097 and NCT01953900) and L1CAM (NCT02311621).[18]

Immune checkpoint inhibitors under investigation include nivolumab (which targets the programed cell death 1/programed cell death ligand 1 axis) in combination with dinutuximab-beta and ^{123}I-MIBG (NCT02914405), pembrolizumab for relapsed neuroblastoma (NCT02332668), and nivolumab with or without the anti-CTLA4 mAb ipilimumab (NCT04500548, NCT02304458, NCT03838042, NCT02914405, NCT04412408 and NCT01445379).[18] Omburtamab is a murine mAb against CD276. Radioimmunotherapy with ^{124}I- or ^{131}I-omburtamab is under investigation for the treatment of CNS malignancies, including neuroblastoma.[21]

Bispecific antibodies that aim to guide T cells to tumor cells include anti-GD2 × anti-CD3 (NCT03860207) and autologous T cells armed with anti-CD3 × naxitamab-gqgk (GD2Bi, NCT02173093). Both are in early-phase clinical trials that include patients with neuroblastoma.[18]

An antineuroblastoma vaccine in the form of a GD2/GD3 conjugate vaccine given subcutaneously with an oral beta-glucan adjuvant is being investigated as part of an early-phase clinical trial at a single institute. The vaccine was administered to patients with high-risk neuroblastoma who had achieved remission after previously relapsing or having progressive disease. The vaccine had a favorable safety profile; however, effects on progression-free survival and OS need further investigation.[22]

Drug delivery systems, gene therapy and virotherapy

Radioactive drug delivery, such as with ^{123}I-MIBG, as a conjugate to other compounds or used alone, may carry radiation directly to tumor cells with minimal harm to normal cells. ^{123}I-MIBG is being evaluated in combination with standard therapy in children with newly-diagnosed high-risk neuroblastoma or ganglioneuroblastoma in the ongoing Phase III COG ANBL1531 trial (NCT03126916). Additionally, omburtamab is being studied in patients with CNS or leptimeningeal metastases (NCT03275402). ^{177}Lutetium-tetraazacyclododecane tetraacetic acid–octreotide is under investigation in a Phase II trial in patients with primary refractory or relapsed high-risk neuroblastoma (NCT04903899).

Nanoparticle- or nanodrug-delivery systems should result in lower systemic side effects, prolonged therapeutic effects and improvements in the pharmacokinetic properties of drugs. Some novel drug-delivery systems use liposomes as carriers.[23] The synthetic retinoid fenretinide, which induces apoptosis in neuroblastoma cell lines, is being evaluated in combination with lenalidomide in delivery systems using nanomicelles as carriers to maximize bioavailability in preclinical models.[24]

Gene therapy has the potential to modulate the undesirable effects of oncogenes by inserting normal genes into the genome. A few studies have been carried out in which viral (usually adenovirus) or non-viral vector-based methods have been used to deliver target genes into neuroblastoma, and gene therapy could potentially be combined with stem cell therapy.[25]

Virotherapy, the use of genetically engineered or naturally occurring viruses that selectively kill cancer cells, is a promising new approach.[26] Virotherapy has been introduced in a few patients with neuroblastoma, for example using autologous mesenchymal stem cells harboring the oncolytic virus Icovir-5, with encouraging results.[27]

Markers for monitoring

Circulating tumor DNA (ctDNA) purified from peripheral blood samples ('liquid biopsy') may allow the detection and characterization of neuroblastoma markers using methods such as digital droplet polymerase chain reaction (ddPCR).[8] For example, low levels of ctDNA have been used in ddPCR assays that have reliably quantified *MYCN* and *ALK* copy numbers, while also estimating allele fractions of specific *ALK* mutants in samples from patients with neuroblastoma.[28]

Long non-coding RNAs (lncRNAs) are a type of RNA with no protein-coding roles that regulate cellular functions (including proliferation, differentiation, cell death, migration and invasion) and the immune response. They have been implicated in the pathogenesis of various malignant cancers including neuroblastoma. Studies defining the roles and mechanisms of lncRNAs in neuroblastoma development have shown that some, such as CAI2, ncRAN, SNHG1, SNHG7, SNHG16, pancEts-1 and NHEG1, behave like oncogenes such that high levels are associated with poor differentiation, advanced disease stage and poor outcome. Other lncRNAs include Paupar, which has a regulatory function in neuroblastoma cell proliferation and differentiation, and XIST, which is highly expressed in neuroblastoma. They may have potential as prognostic biomarkers and could be suitable as drug targets.[13]

MicroRNAs (miRs) are small (19–22 nucleotide) non-coding RNAs involved in gene regulation. OncomiRs, metastamiRs and targeted serum miRs are involved in various cellular processes in cancer, and studies have shown that several oncomiRs (miR-221, miR-181a/b, miR-3934 and miR-223) are highly expressed in neuroblastoma, which correlates with poor prognosis.[13]

Key points – future directions and unmet needs

- There is a lack of treatment options for high-risk patients with neuroblastoma, including options that can be used after the emergence of treatment resistance. Response rates seen with induction chemotherapy are inadequate and useful biomarkers to guide therapy decisions are needed.
- Organizations such as the COG, PEP-CTN, SIOP, NANT consortium and Beat Childhood Cancer research consortium are promoting specific research goals and the coordination of clinical trials in neuroblastoma.
- High-throughput genomic technologies will be crucial to ensure accurate diagnoses for individual patients and to fully personalize therapy.
- Many therapeutic strategies are being developed in clinical trials for neuroblastoma, including therapies targeted against ALK and GD2, and immunotherapies.
- New drug targets and improved and novel technologies for disease monitoring are also emerging.

References

1. Applebaum MA, Desai AV, Glade Bender JL. Emerging and investigational therapies for neuroblastoma. *Expert Opin Orphan Drugs* 2017;5:355–68.
2. Moreno L, Caron H, Geoerger B et al. Accelerating drug development for neuroblastoma – New Drug Development Strategy: an Innovative Therapies for Children with Cancer, European Network for Cancer Research in Children and Adolescents and International Society of Paediatric Oncology Europe Neuroblastoma project. *Expert Opin Drug Discov* 2017; 12:801–11.
3. Castel V, Segura V, Berlanga P. Emerging drugs for neuroblastoma. *Expert Opin Emerg Drugs* 2013;18:155–71.
4. Amoroso L, Erminio G, Makin G et al. Topotecan-vincristine-doxorubicin in stage 4 high-risk neuroblastoma patients failing to achieve a complete metastatic response to rapid COJEC: a SIOPEN study. *Cancer Res Treat* 2018;50:148–55.
5. Johnsen JI, Dyberg C, Fransson S, Wickström M. Molecular mechanisms and therapeutic targets in neuroblastoma. *Pharmacol Res* 2018;131:164–76.

6. Moreno L, Barone G, DuBois SG et al. Accelerating drug development for neuroblastoma: summary of the second Neuroblastoma Drug Development Strategy forum from Innovative Therapies for Children with Cancer and International Society of Paediatric Oncology Europe Neuroblastoma. *Eur J Cancer* 2020;136:52–68.
7. Vassal G, Rousseau R, Blanc P et al. Creating a unique, multi-stakeholder Paediatric Oncology Platform to improve drug development for children and adolescents with cancer. *Eur J Cancer* 2015;51:218–24.
8. Esposito MR, Aveic S, Seydel A, Tonini GP. Neuroblastoma treatment in the post-genomic era. *J Biomed Sci* 2017;24:14.
9. Bosse KR, Maris JM. Advances in the translational genomics of neuroblastoma: from improving risk stratification and revealing novel biology to identifying actionable genomic alterations. *Cancer* 2016;122:20–33.
10. Greengard EG. Molecularly targeted therapy for neuroblastoma. *Children (Basel)* 2018;5:142.
11. Foster JH, Voss SD, Hall DC et al. Activity of crizotinib in patients with ALK-aberrant relapsed/refractory neuroblastoma: a Children's Oncology Group study (ADVL0912). *Clin Cancer Res* 2021;27:3543–8.
12. Fischer M, Moreno L, Ziegler DS et al. Ceritinib in paediatric patients with anaplastic lymphoma kinase-positive malignancies: an open-label, multicentre, phase 1, dose-escalation and dose-expansion study. *Lancet Oncol* 2021;22:1764–76.
13. Aravindan N, Herman T, Aravindan S. Emerging therapeutic targets for neuroblastoma. *Expert Opin Ther Targets* 2020;24:899–914.
14. Joshi S. Targeting the tumor microenvironment in neuroblastoma: recent advances and future directions. *Cancers (Basel)* 2020;12:2057.
15. Phimmachanh M, Han JZR, O'Donnell YEI et al. Histone deacetylases and histone deacetylase inhibitors in neuroblastoma. *Front Cell Dev Biol* 2020;8:578770.
16. Pinto N, DuBois SG, Marachelian A et al. Phase I study of vorinostat in combination with isotretinoin in patients with refractory/recurrent neuroblastoma: a New Approaches to Neuroblastoma Therapy (NANT) trial. *Pediatr Blood Cancer* 2018;65:e27023.
17. DuBois SG, Granger MM, Groshen S et al. Randomized phase II trial of MIBG versus MIBG, vincristine, and irinotecan versus MIBG and vorinostat for patients with relapsed or refractory neuroblastoma: a report from NANT Consortium. *J Clin Oncol* 2021;39:3506–14.

18. Wienke J, Dierselhuis MP, Tytgat GAM et al. The immune landscape of neuroblastoma: challenges and opportunities for novel therapeutic strategies in pediatric oncology. *Eur J Cancer* 2021;144:123–50.
19. Park JA, Cheung NV. Targets and antibody formats for immunotherapy of neuroblastoma. *J Clin Oncol* 2020;38:1836–48.
20. National Cancer Institute. *FDA Approves First Therapy for High-Risk Neuroblastoma*, 2015. cancer.gov/news-events/cancer-currents-blog/2015/dinutuximab-neuroblastoma, last accessed 11 May 2022.
21. Kramer K, Donzelli MA, Pessin MS. Mast cell proliferation in the cerebrospinal fluid after intraventricular administration of anti-B7H3 immunotherapy. *Cancer Immunol Immunother* 2021;70:2411–14.
22. Cheung I, Cheung N, Modak S et al. Survival impact of anti-GD2 antibody response in a Phase II ganglioside vaccine trial among patients with high-risk neuroblastoma with prior disease progression. *J Clin Oncol* 2021;39:215–26.
23. Mobasheri T, Rayzan E, Shabani M et al. Neuroblastoma-targeted nanoparticles and novel nanotechnology-based treatment methods. *J Cell Physiol* 2021;236:1751–75.
24. Orienti I, Nguyen F, Guan P et al. A novel nanomicellar combination of fenretinide and lenalidomide shows marked antitumor activity in a neuroblastoma xenograft model. *Drug Des Devel Ther* 2019;13:4305–19.
25. Kumar MD, Dravid A, Kumar A, Sen D. Gene therapy as a potential tool for treating neuroblastoma – a focused review. *Cancer Gene Ther* 2016;23:115–24.
26. Fukuhara H, Ino Y, Todo T. Oncolytic virus therapy: a new era of cancer treatment at dawn. *Cancer Sci* 2016;107:1373–9.
27. Ruano D, López-Martín JA, Moreno L et al. First-in-human, first-in-child trial of autologous MSCs carrying the oncolytic virus Icovir-5 in patients with advanced tumors. *Mol Ther* 2020;28:1033–42.
28. Peitz C, Sprüssel A, Linke RB et al. Multiplexed quantification of four neuroblastoma DNA targets in a single droplet digital PCR reaction. *J Mol Diagn* 2020;22:1309–23.

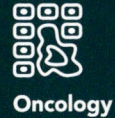

8 Survivorship

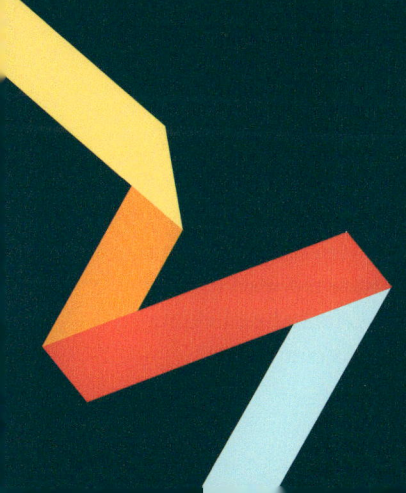

HEALTHCARE

The changing landscape

Survival. For patients with neuroblastoma, 5-year relative survival has increased from 54% among those diagnosed between 1975 and 1984 to 78% between 2005 and 2011,[1] and 5-year survival rates range from 95% in patients with low-risk disease to 50% for those with high-risk disease, a huge increase in the latter group compared with pre-1990 rates.[1,2] As survival improves, the population of long-term survivors has grown, and the long-term morbidity and mortality associated with treatments received in childhood have become more prominent.[3] Better understanding of the long-term morbidities among neuroblastoma survivors is needed to ensure the long-term health of existing survivors, and promote the design of future clinical trials to improve survival and ameliorate late effects.[1]

Late effects. In 2020, it was estimated that nearly 0.5 million long-term survivors of childhood cancer were living in the USA, with survivors experiencing a disproportionately higher frequency of serious medical and psychosocial late effects than the general population.[4] An analysis from the Childhood Cancer Survivor Study (CCSS), a retrospective cohort study that records health information in adults who received a diagnosis of childhood cancer between 1970 and 1986, showed that among 10 937 childhood cancer survivors 30 years after a cancer diagnosis, the cumulative incidence of a chronic health condition was 73.4% (95% CI 69.0, 77.9). Among these survivors, the cumulative incidence of severe, disabling or life-threatening conditions or death due to a chronic condition was 42.4% (95% CI 33.7, 51.2).[5] Although only 4% of the patients in this cohort were initially diagnosed with neuroblastoma, it is likely that as 30-year survivors of neuroblastoma, they initially had low- or intermediate-risk disease.

Late effects were further identified in a CCSS study of neuroblastoma survivors diagnosed between 1970 and 1999 who were found to have increased late mortality. This is likely due to the more intensive treatment received by patients with high-risk neuroblastoma once risk stratification-based therapy regimens were introduced in the later part of this period.[2] Long-term toxicities were reported for up to 95% of this subset of survivors, with toxicities including hearing loss, primary hypothyroidism, ovarian failure, musculoskeletal abnormalities and pulmonary abnormalities in 10% of patients, as well as secondary malignancies. These patients are at relatively high risk of hospitalization.[2]

Late treatment-related morbidities

A wide range of treatment-related late morbidities have been identified, with the type of effect depending on the multiple treatment modalities involved. In recent studies with relatively short follow-up, late effects across a range of categories (Table 8.1) have been found to be caused by radiation exposure (causing secondary malignancy, hypothyroidism or cardiac disease), cisplatin exposure (causing hearing loss or renal dysfunction), alkylating agent exposure (causing renal dysfunction or infertility) and other treatments.[1]

Surgery has been recognized as having the lowest rate of late events. A CCSS study of neuroblastoma survivors (n=954) diagnosed between 1970 and 1986 found that 5-year survivors of neuroblastoma treated with multimodal therapy were 2.2-fold more likely to develop a chronic health condition than those treated with surgery alone.[6]

Induction chemotherapy and myeloablative chemotherapy with ASCT have improved outcomes. During induction, patients typically receive 5–8 cycles of intensive chemotherapy that includes platinum, alkylating and topoisomerase agents.[7] Although the late effects are not yet well defined,[1] a number are known, as are some associated

TABLE 8.1

Prevalence of selected late effects across a range of studies of high-risk neuroblastoma survivors[1]

Late effect	Prevalence (%)
Cardiac	8–20
Pulmonary	19–54
Hypertension/renal	9–63
Abnormal growth	7–100
Gonadal dysfunction	4–83
Hypothyroidism	2–54
Hearing loss	38–92

with radiotherapy. Late effects related to immunotherapy are not yet known and are the subject of ongoing study.

Hearing loss (ototoxicity) is associated with platinum-based chemotherapy. In patients with a history of high-risk disease, its prevalence has been reported to reach 95%. Cisplatin in combination with myeloablative doses of carboplatin increases the risk of hearing loss, which may be compounded by exposure to antibiotics during therapy. Affected survivors of neuroblastoma are at increased risk of learning problems and psychosocial impairments, and should be screened for hearing loss and referred to hearing services as appropriate.[2]

Gonadal dysfunction and infertility are common in patients with childhood cancer who are treated with intensive multimodal therapy. Girls treated with high-dose alkylating agents before ASCT, or with total body irradiation (TBI) or ^{131}I-MIBG therapy, are at increased risk of premature ovarian insufficiency, absent, arrested or delayed puberty, and future infertility, and may require referral to a pediatric endocrinologist for appropriate management. Male patients are also at risk of future infertility. Affected survivors should be made aware of alternative family-building options in a timely fashion, while for females with normal gonadotropins who undergo menarche spontaneously, oocyte or embryo freezing can be considered with input from a reproductive endocrinology specialist.[2]

Renal dysfunction in childhood cancer survivors treated with nephrotoxic therapies, including cisplatin, carboplatin, ifosfamide and radiotherapy involving the kidney region, and/or nephrectomy, has been assessed in multiple studies, with the prevalence of renal adverse effects ranging widely (0–84% across studies). As a result, the risk of renal dysfunction is difficult to quantify with certainty.[8] However, as neuroblastoma survivors often undergo nephrectomy and receive potentially nephrotoxic chemotherapy, radiation to the kidney(s) or potentially nephrotoxic antibiotics, the risk of late renal toxicity is high.[2] Long-term data are lacking and more studies are needed to clarify the risk for late renal toxicity following radiation exposure.[2]

Cardiac disease. Cardiomyopathy, coronary artery disease, pericardial disease, arrhythmias, valvular dysfunction and stroke all contribute to early morbidity and mortality among childhood cancer survivors treated with cardiotoxic therapies such as doxorubicin. In survivors of neuroblastoma, the already elevated risks of congestive heart failure, pericardial disease and valvular abnormalities are further increased 2–5-fold by exposure to anthracyclines, 250 mg/m^2 or more, compared with non-exposed survivors.[9] All survivors should receive careful cardiac follow-up including screening with serial echocardiograms, with any new cardiac symptoms reported to their treating primary care provider.[2]

Pulmonary abnormalities have been identified as a late effect of therapy, particularly among those who have received radiation to the lungs or with high-risk neuroblastoma. In the latter, pulmonary function testing has been reported to show mostly mild-to-moderate chronic respiratory symptoms in 33% of survivors. Busulfan or melphalan prior to ASCT is associated with pulmonary toxicity. Survivors exposed to known pulmonary-toxic chemotherapies should have baseline pulmonary function testing when entering long-term follow-up, with testing repeated as appropriate, and be counseled about smoking avoidance.[2]

Secondary malignancy incidence in survivors of neuroblastoma treated with intensive multimodal therapies is high. One study of patients in clinical trials demonstrated a 10-year cumulative incidence of 1.8% among high-risk patients and 0.38% among low-risk patients, with an 18-fold increase in the frequency of secondary malignancy and a more than 100-fold increase in the frequency of acute myeloid leukemia in high- and intermediate-risk patients compared with the general population.[10] The risk of secondary acute myeloid leukemia or myelodysplastic syndrome increases with the number of dose-intensive chemotherapy cycles received, while there is a possible association between secondary renal cell carcinoma and prior cisplatin exposure. Survivors of neuroblastoma have also been found to have increased risk of secondary biliary adenocarcinoma, chondrosarcoma, genitourinary carcinoma in women, head and neck carcinoma, hepatocellular carcinoma, thyroid papillary carcinoma and melanoma.[2]

Primary hypothyroidism is associated with radiation to the neck, as occurs with TBI, and thyroid dysfunction has also been reported at high rates following ^{131}I-MIBG therapy.[2] Exposed survivors should have annual thyroid function tests and be treated with levothyroxine if primary hypothyroidism is diagnosed.

Growth hormone deficiency is associated with TBI and cranial radiation (with hypothalamic–pituitary doses ≥ 18 Gy) in patients with childhood cancer and can lead to poor linear growth.[2] Growth can also be affected by direct radiation-induced damage to the growth plates of the spine or long bones, which may not respond adequately to growth hormone therapy.[1] Survivors of neuroblastoma with suboptimal linear growth should be referred to an endocrinologist.

Diabetes mellitus is about 7-fold more likely in survivors of neuroblastoma exposed to abdominal radiation than in their siblings, while those treated with TBI are at even greater risk of diabetes and metabolic syndrome. In particular, boys may be less physically active than their peers. Survivors of neuroblastoma who have been exposed to radiotherapy should receive regular counseling about the importance of diet and exercise, and be monitored with fasting blood glucose or hemoglobin A1c tests every 2 years, with referral to a pediatric endocrinologist as appropriate.[2]

Long-term psychological and psychosocial effects. Survivors of neuroblastoma are at increased risk of psychological problems and impaired quality of life. A quality of life-based study of 5-year survivors of neuroblastoma (n = 859; aged < 18 years and diagnosed between 1970 and 1999) found that survivors had higher parent-reported levels of antisocial behavior, anxiety and/or depression, attention deficits, headstrong behavior, and peer conflict or social withdrawal than their siblings (all $p ≤ 0.01$). Moreover, the presence of pulmonary disease was associated with impairment in all five domains ($p < 0.01$), and psychological impairment was associated with increased use of special education services and low educational attainment.[11] Other studies using self-report questionnaires have found that survivors of neuroblastoma have increased scores for poor emotional health, lower individual and household incomes, and having never been employed or married, suggesting decreased social integration.[2] Given the risk of long-term psychological and psychosocial effects in survivors of neuroblastoma, there is strong evidence that survivors should undergo formal neuropsychological testing to allow timely educational support where needed.

COG surveillance guidelines for survivors and investigations into late effects

The COG Long-Term Follow-Up Guidelines for survivors of childhood, adolescent and young adult cancers are a resource for healthcare professionals who provide ongoing care to survivors of pediatric malignancies.[12] They comprise risk-based, exposure-related clinical practice guidelines for the screening and management of late effects resulting from therapies used during the treatment of pediatric malignancies, and are appropriate for asymptomatic survivors of childhood, adolescent or young adult cancers presenting for routine medical follow-up. They aim to:
- provide recommendations for screening and management of late effects that may potentially arise because of treatment for childhood cancer
- increase awareness of potential late effects
- standardize and enhance follow-up care provided to survivors.[12]

Late effects in high-risk neuroblastoma survivors as a result of modern regimens and exposures (including the use of induction chemotherapy and ASCT, radiotherapy, chemotherapy, *cis*-retinoic acid, immunotherapy and ^{123}I-MIBG), including secondary malignancies, are the subject of long-term study by the COG.

The COG Neuroblastoma Biology study (ANBL00B1; NCT00904241) has recruited more than 700 high-risk neuroblastoma patients who were treated between 2000 and 2011, and aims to recruit around 10 000 patients in total.

The COG Late Effects After High-Risk Neuroblastoma (LEAHRN) study (ALTE 15N2; NCT03057626) opened in 2016. It has recruited around 400 survivors to characterize late effects, assess predictors and possible biomarkers of these late effects, and identify factors predictive of health-related quality of life.

Key points – survivorship

- The population of long-term survivors of neuroblastoma has grown, and an understanding of the long-term morbidities among survivors is needed to ensure their continuing good health.
- Late effects include hearing loss, gonadal dysfunction and infertility, pulmonary abnormalities, cardiac disease, renal dysfunction, diabetes, hypothyroidism, secondary malignancy, growth hormone deficiency, and psychological and psychosocial issues.
- COG Long-Term Follow-Up Guidelines are available for healthcare professionals who support survivors of pediatric malignancies.
- Late effects following modern treatments for neuroblastoma are the subject of ongoing studies.

References

1. Speleman F, Park JR, Henderson TO. Neuroblastoma: a tough nut to crack. *Am Soc Clin Oncol Educ Book* 2016;35:e548–57.
2. Friedman DN, Henderson TO. Late effects and survivorship issues in patients with neuroblastoma. *Children (Basel)* 2018;5:107.
3. Robison LL, Armstrong GT, Boice JD et al. The Childhood Cancer Survivor Study: a National Cancer Institute-supported resource for outcome and intervention research. *J Clin Oncol* 2009;27:2308–18.
4. Chow EJ, Ness KK, Armstrong GT et al. Current and coming challenges in the management of the survivorship population. *Semin Oncol* 2020;47:23–39.
5. Oeffinger KC, Mertens AC, Sklar CA et al. Chronic health conditions in adult survivors of childhood cancer. *N Engl J Med* 2006;355:1572–82.
6. Laverdière C, Liu Q, Yasui Y et al. Long-term outcomes in survivors of neuroblastoma: a report from the Childhood Cancer Survivor Study. *J Natl Cancer Inst* 2009;101:1131–40.

7. Smith V, Foster J. High-risk neuroblastoma treatment review. *Children (Basel)* 2018;5:114.
8. Knijnenburg SL, Mulder RL, Schouten-Van Meeteren AYN et al. Early and late renal adverse effects after potentially nephrotoxic treatment for childhood cancer. *Cochrane Database Syst Rev* 2013;10:CD008944.
9. Mulrooney DA, Yeazel MW, Kawashima T et al. Cardiac outcomes in a cohort of adult survivors of childhood and adolescent cancer: retrospective analysis of the Childhood Cancer Survivor Study cohort. *BMJ* 2009;339:b4606.
10. Applebaum MA, Vaksman Z, Lee SM et al. Neuroblastoma survivors are at increased risk for second malignancies: a report from the International Neuroblastoma Risk Group Project. *Eur J Cancer* 2017;72:177–85.
11. Zheng DJ, Krull KR, Chen Y et al. Long-term psychological and educational outcomes for survivors of neuroblastoma: a report from the Childhood Cancer Survivor Study. *Cancer* 2018;124:3220–30.
12. Children's Oncology Group. *COG Long-Term Follow-Up Guidelines for Survivors of Childhood, Adolescent, and Young Adult Cancers, Version 5.0*, 2018. childrensoncologygroup.org/ survivorshipguidelines, last accessed 11 May 2022.

Useful resources

Alex's Lemonade Stand Foundation
for Childhood Cancer
alexslemonade.org

Beat Childhood Cancer Research
Consortium
research.beatcc.org

Children's Neuroblastoma Cancer
Foundation
cncfhope.org

Children's Oncology Group
childrensoncologygroup.org

International Society of Paediatric
Oncology (SIOP)
siop-online.org

New Approaches to Neuroblastoma
Therapy (NANT) consortium
nant.org

Pediatric Early Phase Clinical Trials
Network (PEP-CTN)
ctep.cancer.gov/initiativesPrograms/
pep-ctn.htm

St Baldrick's Foundation
stbaldricks.org

FastTest

You've read the book ... now test yourself with key questions from the authors

- Go to the FastTest for this title
  FREE at **karger.com/fastfacts**
- Approximate time **10 minutes**
- For best retention of the key issues, try taking the FastTest before and after reading

Index

abdominal tumors 28, 44, 53, 54–5
adrenal tumors 14, 18, 31
adverse effects
 chemotherapy 61, 63, 97–9
 dinutuximab 63–4
 late effects 96–102
 ^{131}I-MIBG 65–6, 100
 radiotherapy 98, 100
 surgery 55
age 10–11
ALK and ALK 20–1, 23, 48
ALK inhibitors 48, 61, 86
aneuploidy 14, 21–2, 33, 48
angiogenesis (as target) 87
antibiotics 67
ASCT (autologous stem cell transplant) 62–3, 65
ATRX 23

Beat Childhood Cancer Research Consortium 83
bevacizumab 87
biomarkers 21–2, 83, 91
biopsy 33, 36, 53
bispecific antibodies 90
'blueberry muffin' effect 30
bone metastases 29, 36–7, 61

CAR T-cell therapy 66, 89
cardiac disease 99
catecholamines 33

central hypoventilation syndrome 14
central venous catheters 67
ceritinib 86
cervical tumors 28, 44, 54
chemotherapy 56, 58–9, 60–3, 64, 66, 68–9, 82–3
 adverse effects 61, 63, 97–9
Children's Oncology Group (COG) 83, 101
chromosomal abnormalities 14, 21–2, 33, 48
cisplatin 98
clinical presentation 28–31, 32, 56
clinical trials 12, 83–90
congenital tumors 14, 31–2, 56–7
copy number variations 14, 22, 33
cost of healthcare 77
crizotinib 48, 61, 86
CT imaging 35
ctDNA 91
Curie scoring system 36, 37–8, 62
cytopenia 32, 65

diabetes mellitus 100
diagnosis 28–38
 age at 10
 delayed 76, 78
 differentials 31, 32
 imaging 31, 32, 34–6
 lab tests 32–4
 overdiagnosis 11
 presentation 28–31, 32, 56
 staging 36–8

dinutuximab 61, 63–4, 89
dinutuximab-beta 63
DNA, tumor (ctDNA) 91
drug delivery systems 90

eflornithine 64
environmental causes 13
epidemiology 10–13, 14, 76
epigenetics 87–8
ethnicity 11, 13, 76–7
etiology 13–14

familial disease 13–14, 23
follow-up 67, 101

GD2 antibodies 61, 63–4, 66, 89, 90
gender 11
gene therapy 90–1
genetics 13–14, 21–4, 48
 tests 33, 85, 91
geography 11–12
gonadal dysfunction 98
gross total resection (GTR) 54–5
growth hormone deficiency 100

health disparities 11–12, 13, 76–9
hearing loss 98
hematology 32
hepatic metastases 29, 53
high-risk tumors 13, 46–7
 and ethnicity/SES 76, 77–8
 late effects 97, 99, 101
 management 53–5, 59–68, 69, 82–3

107

Hirschsprung disease 14
histology 33–4
histone deacetylase
 (HDAC) inhibitors 88
history taking 32
Homer Wright pseudo-
 rosettes 33
hypothyroidism 100

imaging 31, 32, 34–6, 44
immune checkpoint
 inhibitors 89
immunization 67
 anti-tumor 90
immunohistochemistry
 21, 34
immunotherapy 61,
 63–4, 66, 87, 88–90
incidence 10–12
infants 10, 32, 46–7, 56–7
infertility 98
INRG risk-classification
 system 43–8
INRGSS (staging system)
 42–3
INSS (staging system) 42
intermediate-risk tumors
 management 53, 58–9,
 67, 68
 risk status 46–7
International Society of
 Paediatric Oncology
 83–4
ipilimumab 89
irinotecan 64, 66
isotretinoin 66

kidney dysfunction 54,
 98

late effects 96–102
liver metastases 29, 53
lncRNA 91
location of tumors 18, 28
long-term effects 96–102
lorlatinib 87

low-risk tumors
 management 43, 52–3,
 57–8, 68
 risk status 46–7
lung disease 99
lymph nodes 29, 42, 54

management 52–69
 chemotherapy 56, 58–9,
 60–3, 64, 66, 82–3,
 97–9
 follow-up 67, 101
 high-risk tumors 53–5,
 59–68, 82–3
 immunotherapy 61,
 63–4, 66, 87, 88–90
 intermediate-risk
 tumors 6, 53, 58–9,
 67
 late effects 96–102
 limitations 82–3
 low-risk tumors 43,
 52–3, 57–8
 ^{131}I/^{123}I-MIBG 61, 65–6,
 88, 90, 100
 MS stage 53, 57
 OMAS 31
 palliative 67–8
 paraspinal tumors 56
 perinatal 56–7
 radiotherapy 55–6, 59,
 63, 98, 100
 refractory/relapsed
 disease 64–6, 68,
 82–3, 87, 88
 research 85–91
 surgery 52–5, 56, 97
mediastinal tumors 28,
 44, 54
metastasis 29, 36–8,
 45, 47
 MS stage 47, 53, 57
MIBG
 scintigraphy (^{123}I) 36–8
 therapy (^{123}I/^{131}I) 61,
 65–6, 88, 90, 100
microRNA 91
microscopy 33–4

MRI (magnetic
 resonance imaging)
 31, 35–6
mutations 14, 21–4, 48
MYCN and MYC-N 14,
 20, 22, 23
 and risk status 43,
 45, 48
 as a target 86

nanoparticles 90
naxitamab-gqgk 61, 66,
 89, 90
neck tumors 28, 44, 54
nerve growth factor
 19–20
neural crest 18–19
Neuroblastoma New
 Drug Development
 Strategy 84
neurofibromatosis 14
New Approaches to
 Neuroblastoma
 Therapy (NANT) 83
nivolumab 89
NRAS 24

omburtamab 89, 90
oncogenesis 18–24
opsoclonus-
 myoclonus-ataxia
 syndrome (OMAS)
 29–31
ornithine decarboxylase
 inhibitors 87
ototoxicity 98
ovarian dysfunction 98
overdiagnosis 11

palliative care 67–8
paraneoplastic
 syndromes 29–31
paraspinal tumors 28,
 44, 56, 68
pathogenesis 18–24
pazopanib 87

Index

Pediatric Early Phase Clinical Trials Network 83
Pediatric Oncology Platform 84–5
pembrolizumab 89
perinatal disease 14, 31–2, 56–7
personalized medicine 85
PHOX2B and PHOX2B 14, 21
physical examination 28–31, 32
poverty 11–12, 77–8
prenatal diagnosis 31
prevalence 10
prognosis 12–13, 43–9
genetics 21, 22, 48
psychosocial effects of treatment 100–1
PTNP11 23
pulmonary disease 99

raccoon eyes 30
race 11, 13, 76–7
radiography 34
radiopharmaceuticals (^{123}I/^{131}I-MIBG)
diagnostic 36–8
therapeutic 61, 65–6, 88, 90, 100
radiotherapy 55–6, 59, 63, 98, 100
refractory/relapsed disease 64–6, 68, 82–3, 87, 88
regression, spontaneous 20, 53, 56

renal dysfunction 54, 98
repotrectinib 86–7
research
late effects in survivors 101
treatment 83–92
retinoids 63, 90
risk stratification 12–13, 43–9, 85
RNA markers 91

scintigraphy 36–8
screening programs 11
secondary malignancies 99
segmental chromosome aberrations 22, 48
sex 11
side effects see adverse effects
site of tumors 18, 28
skeletal metastases 29, 36–7, 61
skin metastases 29
'small round blue cells' 33–4
social support 78
socioeconomic status 11–12, 77–9
spine see paraspinal tumors
staging 36–8, 42–3, 49
INRG risk-classification 43–8
stem cell transplantation 62–3, 65
surgery 52–5, 56, 68, 97

surveillance 67, 101
see also watchful waiting
survival rates 12–13, 82, 96
differences in 13, 76, 77, 78
survivorship 96–102
symptoms 28–9, 30–1, 56

targeted therapies 61, 63–4, 66, 86–90
temozolomide 64, 66
temsirolimus 64
TERT 22
thoracic tumors 28, 44, 54
thyroid disease 100
TP53 24
transcription factors 20–1
transportation 78
treatment see management
tyrosine kinase (ALK) inhibitors 48, 61, 86

ultrasonography 35

vaccination 67
anti-tumor 90
vasoactive intestinal peptide syndrome 31
virotherapy 91
vorinostat 88

watchful waiting 43, 56, 57, 58

X-rays 34